Reimagine Well Learn Guide:

Adolescent and Young Adult (AYA) Cancer

From Diagnosis To Wellbeing

Martin Casella

Roger Holzberg

Adele Sender

If you, or someone you love, has been diagnosed with cancer and you are between the ages of 15 and 39, this Adolescent and Young Adult (AYA) Learn Guide will help you through the anxiety of a cancer diagnosis. Our goal is to provide you with concise, evidence-based, easily understood educational resources throughout your entire cancer journey.

With links to online resources, this book will serve to empower both patients and caregivers navigating from diagnosis to wellbeing. It will also provide you with a (private and safe) support community to connect with, where you can learn from the cancer survivors and families, who have gone before you.

— Team Reimagine Well

ISBN: 978-0-9992364-3-7

NOTE:

Both parts of this book are designed to go hand-in-hand. We strongly encourage you to read forward only to the phase you are in right at this moment:

- Diagnosis
- Treatment
- Healing
- Wellbeing

As you utilize Part 1 of the Learn Guide to educate yourself, and get coached on how to become an empowered patient, you may also want to begin creating your support community. That AYA Support Community can be accessed at http://www.reimaginewellcommunity.com/, and the details on how to best use it are found in Part 2 of this Learn Guide.

A message to you newly diagnosed adolescent and young adult cancer patients… and your families. From Leonard Sender, M.D, one of the Founders of Reimagine Well.

"Information can lead to knowledge. Knowledge is power. You have to become empowered to learn, then ask the right questions and get the information you need. The best way to get the type of treatment that is right for you, that will lead to the type of outcome we want for you, is to become fully engaged in the process."

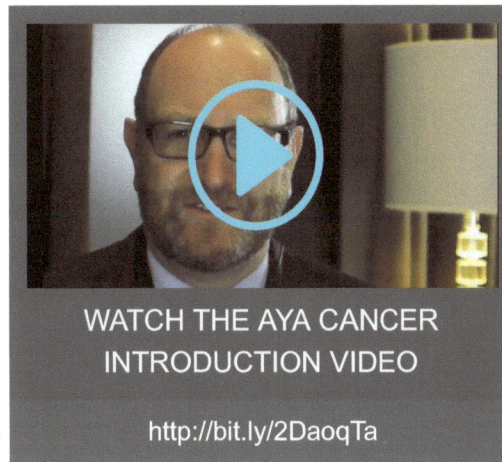

WATCH THE AYA CANCER
INTRODUCTION VIDEO

http://bit.ly/2DaoqTa

After you download this Enhanced eBook onto your phone, tablet, computer, or print a hard copy, bring it with you to all meetings with your Healthcare Professionals.

— Team Reimagine Well

"Never believe statistics. Statistics are based on everybody else. You're your own individual. You are your own person. I brought hope with me to the hospital. You can't do anything without hope!"
— AYA Cancer Patient,
Age 17, Medulloblastoma Brain Cancer

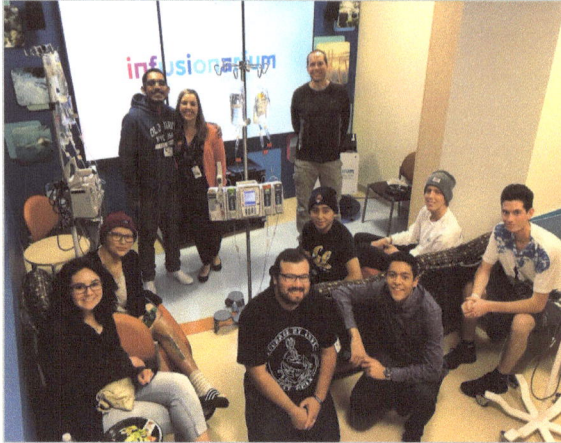

"What an amazing opportunity to build a community and connect with people who can relate to what it feels like when you're told you have cancer… in the end, the experience of being more transparent with my fears was cathartic and healing."
— AYA Cancer Patient,
Age 23, Colon Cancer

"It helps to share information and hope. I totally agree that keeping positive and never giving up hope is paramount."
— AYA Cancer Caregiver/Dad

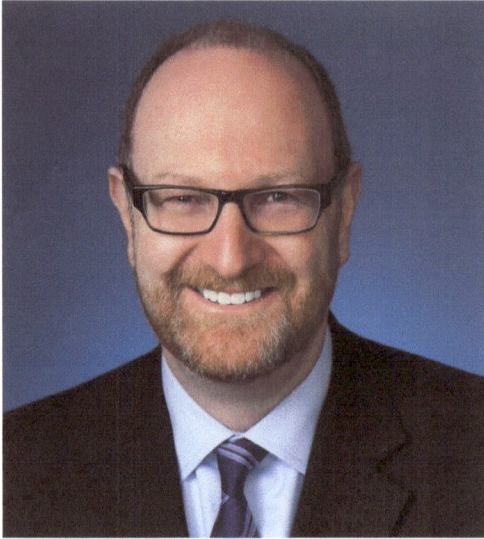

Leonard Sender, M.D.

Dr. Leonard "Lennie" Sender is a pioneer in cancer care treatment, especially in adolescents and young adults, which are typically underrepresented cohorts in oncological research. Dr. Sender is Director of the Adolescent and Young Adult (AYA) Cancer Program at CHOC Children's in Orange County, where he leads one of the nation's largest programs considering the unique challenges faced by AYA cancer patients, such as preservation of fertility, management of the effects of treatment, and the psychosocial impact of the disease. As an innovative leader in research, Dr. Sender is conducting extensive studies to improve outcomes and quality of life for AYAs. He is Chairman Emeritus of the Stupid Cancer organization and is a founding member and chairman of SeventyK.org, an advocacy site for AYAs with cancer.

Dr. Sender received his medical education in South Africa and his pediatric internship and residency at UC Irvine Medical Center. His pediatric hematology/oncology subspecialty training included Children's Hospital of Los Angeles.

"I've been involved with pediatric cancers, adolescents, and young adults for 30 years. The thing I want to say to a patient who has just completed their treatment is, firstly, congratulations and, secondly, well done. What we need to talk about now is how we get you to your new normal, how we get you to adulthood, how we understand all the consequences of the therapy that you've been through, and how we make sure that you truly have wellbeing going forward."

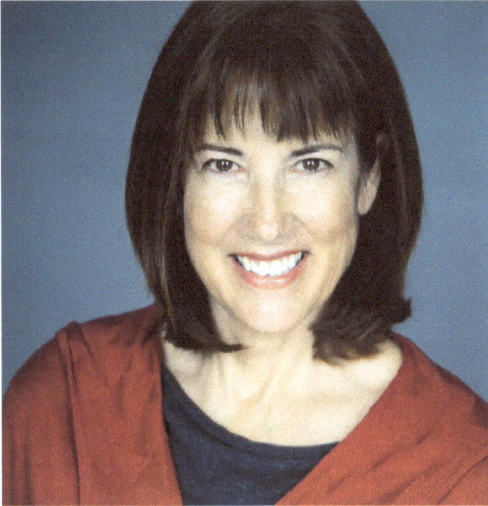

Jocelyn Harrison, MPH, RD

Jocelyn Harrison received her Master of Public Health from UCLA and completed a dietetic internship at the Los Angeles Veterans Hospital. She has developed nutrition programs and marketing for the USDA Dietary Guidelines for Americans, Choose Health LA, and the American Diabetes Association. Her Reimagine Well work includes literature reviews and helping with "immersive healing environment" patient benefit studies.

"The most important things you can do to fight cancer and prepare yourself for treatment are - eat a mostly plant-based diet, maintain a healthy weight and be physically active. Although a diagnosis can be overwhelming, you have a part to play in your own treatment. Be empowered, this is your journey."

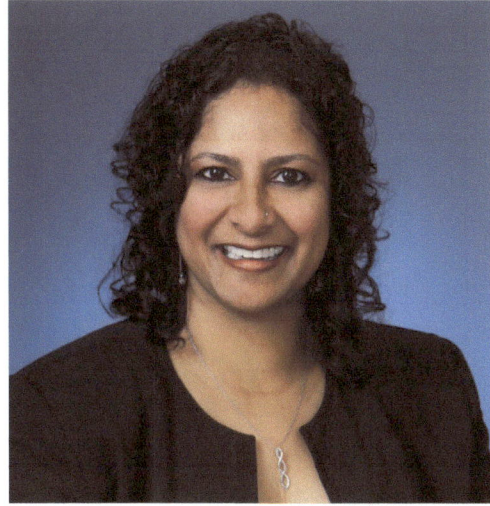

Jenee Areeckal, MSW, LCSW

Jenee Areeckal is a clinical social worker at UCSF Benioff Children's Hospital. She is a three-time cancer survivor and an amputee due to osteogenic sarcoma who knows what it is like to live through and be treated for cancer as a teen and young adult. Today she uses her story to inspire her patients and families both during and after treatment. She is proof that life after cancer can be wonderful and fulfilling.

"I am a three time AYA cancer survivor. I had osteogenic sarcoma when I was 15, with two relapses, and had ovarian cancer at 38. I've been taking care of teens and young adults with cancer for about 10 years. It's been my life's passion to help them navigate through not only their treatment, but also post-cancer Survivorship. It's also very important for me to help educate patients how to become strong survivors. I hope that by seeing me "get busy living", patients have hope that it is possible to survive and thrive after cancer."

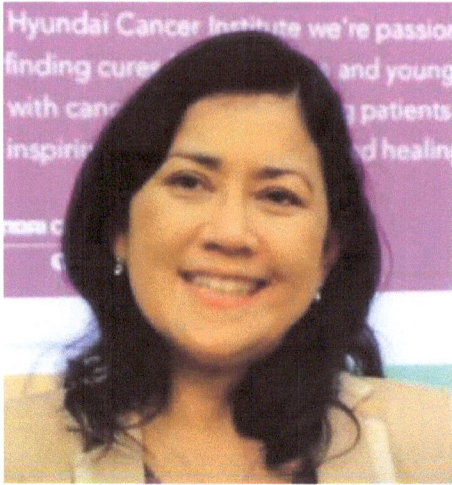

Lilibeth Torno, M.D.

Dr. Lilibeth Torno serves as Assistant Division Chief of Oncology as well as Clinical Director of the Cancer Institute Outpatient Services and the ACTS (After Cancer Treatment survivorship) program at CHOC Children's Hospital. She recently pioneered the development of a multi-institutional pediatric and AYA cancer survivorship consortium in Southern California as a research collaboration platform for cancer survivorship.

Dr. Torno completed her fellowship training at Children's Hospital of Los Angeles. She completed her residency at CHOC CHildren's. She attended medical school at University of Santo Tomas, Manila, Philippines.

"I've been involved with pediatric cancers, adolescents, and young adults for 30 years. The thing I want to say to a patient who has just completed their treatment is, firstly, congratulations and, secondly, well done. What we need to talk about now is how we get you to your new normal, how we get you to adulthood, how we understand all the consequences of the therapy that you've been through, and how we make sure that you truly have wellness going forward."

Diagnosis

Take A Deep Breath

The Diagnosis Phase - What Is AYA Cancer?

"AYA cancer is cancer that affects adolescents and young adults (ages 15-39). A positive attitude is crucial in dealing with AYA cancer. Know that there is great research going on currently and people survive this every day."

— Leonard Sender, M.D.

Seventy thousand Americans aged 15 to 39 years old are diagnosed with AYA cancer every year. To put that in perspective, it's about six times the number of cancers diagnosed in children ages 0-14.

Cancer in adolescents and young adults manifests like a different disease than cancers seen in children or older adults. While a great deal more medical research is needed to achieve better survival outcomes in AYA patients, there's a link below to many articles about current research. As you read on through the diagnosis phase of the Learn Guide, you'll start with a list of the most common AYA cancers. Then you'll move along through information about other issues that may directly affect you after your diagnosis. This includes topics such as prognosis, second opinions, fertility preservation and nutrition.

"After being diagnosed, I was instructed to go back to school (freshman year). After my surgery I recovered at the end of March and began normal classes. I was told I wouldn't need chemotherapy, but within a few days they changed their mind… I began chemo …it sucked. I lost all my hair and still experienced panic attacks. But they helped me get through it. I have the most amazing oncologist… she has become my family. I trust her with my entire LIFE! Also an inspiring social worker… And my amazing family and friends. YOU ARE NOT ALONE!"

— AYA Cancer Patient, Age 26, Testicular Cancer

TO LEARN MORE

See a snapshot of adolescent and young adult cancers at www.cancer.gov/types/aya

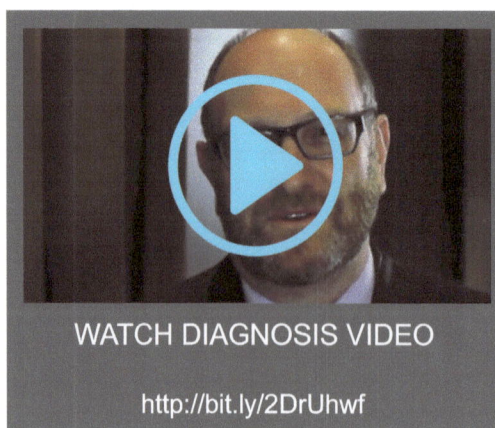

WATCH DIAGNOSIS VIDEO

http://bit.ly/2DrUhwf

"When a patient is diagnosed with cancer, the world stops for them… time is shattered… everything they ever thought they were going to do with their life suddenly comes to a crashing stop…"
— Leonard Sender, M.D.

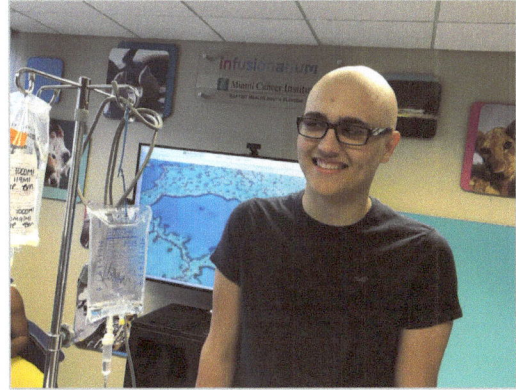

The Most Common AYA Cancers

It is very important for you, your family and your caregivers to know exactly what kind of cancer you have. Here is just a few:

- Breast Cancer
- Brain Tumors
- Cervical Cancer
- Colorectal Cancer

- Germ Cell Tumors
- Leukemia
- Liver Cancer

- Lymphoma
- Melanoma
- Sarcoma

What's The First Thing I Should Do?

The first thing to do, after you take that deep breath (whether you are a patient or a caregiver) is to start putting together your Care Team.

You should ask many questions to these various practitioners before you make up your mind about which of them are the best choices for you. As an AYA cancer patient, there is a health campaign about which you, your family and your caregivers should know.

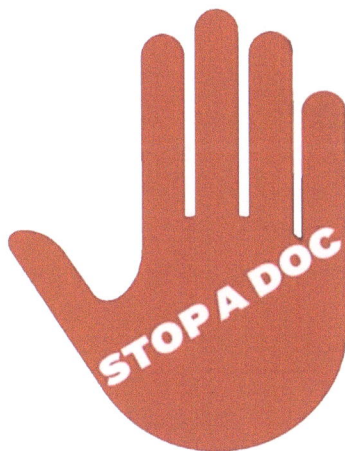

It's called Stop A Doc! This campaign will help you ask the right questions to make sure you get the right doctor and the right treatment. As a AYA cancer patient, you may be interested in having children at some point. If so - along with asking about your treatment's impact on your reproductive chances in the future - you need to talk to your doctor about fertility preservation. Unless you've discussed fertility preservation, make sure the treatment you are about to undergo won't harm your ability to have children.

Here are the five questions that Stop A Doc! recommends you ask your doctor. After you read through them, there's a link at the end of this section for more info.

1. Do you know there's an adolescent and young adult cancer segment called AYA?
2. Are you aware of the unique physical, psychological and social needs of AYA cancer patients?
3. Do you know if there are any available clinical trials for AYA patients?
4. Can you refer AYA patients to any AYA specific resources?
5. Do you treat AYA patients and if so, do you have academic and clinical experience treating 15 to 39-year-old cancer patients.

Make Sure You're Sure

After the discussion following these questions, if you or your caregiver feels reluctant about working with this doctor, follow your instincts. Get out of there! Find someone else with whom you feel more comfortable. It's your treatment. And your life.

> "No question is silly. Ask your doctors, nurses, everyone…anything you can think of!"
> — AYA Cancer Patient, Age 19, Leukemia

Second Opinions

After your doctor gives you advice about your diagnosis and treatment plan, you may want to get another doctor's opinion before you begin treatment. This is known as getting a second opinion. You do this by asking another specialist—someone at a good, reputable university hospital or well-known medical center—to review all of the materials related to your case. A second opinion doctor can confirm or suggest modifications to your original doctor's proposed treatment plan. This doctor can also provide reassurance that you have explored all your options, and answer any other questions you may have.

> "The moment I met my doctor, I knew he was the one. He made us feel very comfortable . He wanted to know all about me, my family and especially what I was feeling. Faith in your doctor is key!"
> — AYA Cancer Patient, Age 27, Thyroid Cancer

TO LEARN MORE

Help With Finding A Doctor: https://www.cancer.gov/about-cancer/managing-care/services/doctor-facility-fact-sheet

Stop A Doc: http://seventyk.org/get-involved/stop-a-doc

Definition of Fertility Preservation: https://www.cancer.gov/publications/dictionaries/cancer-terms?cdrid=732564

SeventyK Fertility Preservation: http://seventyk.org/get-educated/fertility-preservation

Definition of Clinical Trials: https://www.cancer.gov/publications/dictionaries/cancer-terms?CdrID=45961

What Are The Differences Between Practitioners?

You are going to hear a lot of new and unfamiliar medical terms. Below are a few of the Practitioners you may be dealing with.

ONCOLOGIST

An oncologist tends to the medical side of treatment, and will take care of your whole body and health during chemotherapy and radiation treatment.

SURGEON

A surgeon will operate on you if you need to have a tumor removed.

RADIATION ONCOLOGIST

A radiation oncologist will be the one to perform any radiation procedures needed to kill cancer cells.

RADIOLOGIST

A radiologist performs and reviews the scans needed to determine where the cancer is and how it's growing or changing.

REGISTERED DIETITIAN

A registered dietitian has special training in the use of diet and nutrition to keep the body healthy. As part of your medical team, RDs are skilled, competent and knowledgeable in how to provide safe and effective nutrition to improve your overall health. An RD who works with cancer patients may also be called an ONCOLOGY NUTRITIONIST.

ONCOLOGY SOCIAL WORKER

An oncology social worker helps patients, families, and caregivers deal with the experience of facing cancer.

What Treatment Options Do I Have?

SURGERY

The surgeon will remove any tumors the oncologist decides are necessary and pertinent to remove.

MORE INFO ON SURGERY: Surgery: https://childrensoncologygroup.org/index.php/treatmentoptions/surgery

RADIATION THERAPY

The radiation oncologist would begin treating you with radiation therapy in combination with hormone therapy if that is needed as well.

MORE INFO ON RADIATION THERAPY: https://childrensoncologygroup.org/index.php/treatmentoptions/radiationtherapy

CHEMOTHERAPY

Sometimes, you may need all three treatment options: a surgeon to remove tumors, an oncologist to treat your whole body, and a radiation oncologist to treat you with radiation therapy and chemotherapy.

MORE INFO ON CHEMOTHERAPY: https://childrensoncologygroup.org/index.php/treatmentoptions/chemotherapy

IMMUNOTHERAPY

The new form of cancer care is to harness our own immune systems. Chemo and radiation are used at lower doses. That combination is enhanced with the body's immune cells to kill and control the cancer. This allows patients to be treated without the long-term toxic effects of radiation and chemo.

MORE INFO ON IMMUNOTHERAPY: https://childrensoncologygroup.org/index.php/treatmentoptions/immunotherapy

ALTERNATIVE TREATMENTS

Complementary and alternative are terms used to describe products, practices, and systems not part of mainstream medicine. They are called "complementary" when they are used with your medical treatment. They are called "alternative" when they are used instead of proven or standard medical treatments.

MORE INFO ON ALTERNATE TREATMENTS: https://nccih.nih.gov/health/integrative-health#integrative

> "I totally agree that keeping positive and never giving up is paramount"
> — AYA Cancer Caregiver/Brother

TO LEARN MORE
Radiation: http://bit.ly/1tWflhN
Chemotherapy: http://bit.ly/1roCBZB
Immunotherapy: http://bit.ly/2jqAhUw
Alternative Treatments: http://bit.ly/2jqgCDV

How Should I Think About Prognosis?

THE EXACT KIND OF CANCER AND STAGING

You need to understand the exact cancer you have and the exact stage you are in. Once you have a Care Team you are happy with, you need to discuss and process this information with them.

STATISTIC BASED PROGNOSIS

Get a statistic based prognosis based on your current stage. Remember - these are just statistics.

GET THE FACTS

Ask your doctor not to "Dumb it Down." You want the facts!

A GUIDELINE

Not all data will apply to you, but it can give you a guideline for what will happen if you choose different options during your treatment. For more help, and a better understanding of how this part of the diagnosis phase works, have a look at the articles below, along with the series of videos made by the National Cancer Institute.

TO LEARN MORE

Understanding Cancer Prognosis: http://www.cancer.gov/about-cancer/diagnosis-staging/prognosis
NCI Prognosis Video Series: https://www.cancer.gov/about-cancer/diagnosis-staging/prognosis#video-series

Where Do I Learn?

Be careful about using information from undocumented websites and companies that are not real medical advisors. This warning also applies to well-meaning family and friends without medical training and/or experience with serious cancer issues. Seek out licensed, Board-certified medical practitioners.

> "What I really wanted to hear was what had worked for people just like me… yesterday!"
> — AYA Cancer Patient, Age 37, Ovarian Cancer

TO LEARN MORE

National Cancer Institute: https://www.cancer.gov/
American Cancer Society: https://www.cancer.org/
Children's Oncology Group: https://childrensoncologygroup.org/
American Institute of Cancer Research: http://www.aicr.org/

How Quickly Should I Move Forward?

Some AYA cancers grow very rapidly. So many AYA patients don't have the luxury of time to process their diagnoses, find the right doctor and begin treatment. There is a condition called "analysis paralysis." It's when you think too much about what medical decision to make next. Don't let your tumor grow as you're debating what to do. Focus on finding a doctor you trust and then decide on a treatment option.

Preserving Fertility

For AYA patients, fertility preservation is particularly important. Some of the cancer treatments you may receive could actually impair your ability to have children in the future. Before you go through your cancer treatment, you should consider your various fertility preservation options. Your options will depend on your diagnosis and treatment plan, and the location of the cancer. Making a careful decision about which option to use now will optimize the options you have after your treatment.

During the diagnosis phase you may be under time constraints to make momentous decisions about your future fertility and your reproductive choices. If you have an aggressive disease, your oncologist might want to initiate chemotherapy or radiation quickly. You might have to make very big decisions in a very short period of time.

Your choices may include:

- For males who have gone through puberty, the most widely used and reliable fertility preservation method is sperm banking.
- Males who have not gone through puberty are not yet producing sperm, so research is focused on using frozen testicular tissue.
- For females who have gone through puberty we can freeze eggs or embryos, or try experimental ovarian tissue transplants.
- Females who have not begun menstruating can be candidates for ovarian tissue cryopreservation (freezing).

TO LEARN MORE

American Society for Reproductive Medicine: http://bit.ly/2y6xRgQ

Definition of Fertility Preservation: http://bit.ly/2wFF6KP

Definition of Puberty: https://www.cancer.gov/publications/dictionaries/cancer-terms?cdrid=440113

Definition of Sperm Banking: https://www.cancer.gov/publications/dictionaries/cancer-terms?cdrid=43974

Definition of Testicular Tissue Banking: https://www.cancer.gov/publications/dictionaries/cancer-terms?cdrid=779599

Definition of Egg Cryopreservation: https://www.cancer.gov/publications/dictionaries/cancer-terms?cdrid=732567

Definition of Ovarian Tissue Banking: https://www.cancer.gov/publications/dictionaries/cancer-terms?CdrID=779590

Definition of Ovarian Cryopreservation:https://www.cancer.gov/publications/dictionaries/cancer-terms?cdrid=774381

"Coming Out" In Public/Who Should I Tell?

"I suggest you tell the world." — Leonard Sender, M.D.

As Dr. Sender puts it: "There is nothing worse than for a cancer patient to feel alone. I think you need to tell your family, your friends, your loved ones… talk to and tell people who've been through it before. What are the tips they have?"

That said, you need to move at your own pace, you need to share the information with people you trust, people who will be supportive and people who will be there for you. A cancer patient may need to be careful about whom he or she tells during the diagnosis, treatment and healing phases - just because there is always so much information that may need to be shared with so many other people. During these times it is often helpful to ask a close family member or friend to be a gateway to all the others for your frequent or occasional medical updates At the heart of Dr. Sender's statement is a huge piece of advice: tell people so that you are not alone.

Social Media and Blogging

As important as it is to tell your family, your friends and your loved ones about your cancer diagnosis, you might want to put the brakes on when it comes to sharing the information - specifically the details - on social media platforms such as Facebook, Instagram, Reddit, Twitter and whatever new platform pops up tomorrow. Sometimes there is such a thing as TMI - Too Much Information. At a certain point you will lose control over who and how people learn about your condition. That may interfere with - or cause a situation - at school or at work. Just proceed with caution and care. Get advice from others who've been there.

Blogging about what you're going through medically is a different situation. And participating in online chat rooms and private groups that have been formed by other cancer patients is actually a very good thing. It gives you a place to be with your tribe. It gives you an opportunity to blow off some steam, to be emotional. Just remember there is very little privacy left now in the world. And there are some details of what you are going through that you might just want to save for yourself, your family, your close friends and relatives, and your Care Team.

"Participating in the Reimagine Well support community gives me the opportunity to know that I'm not alone, that there are other(s)... experiencing it in real-time. From them I can learn something, and maybe contribute to others in return."
— AYA Cancer Patient, Age 26, Breast Cancer

Nutrition And Active Lifestyle During This Phase

"The most important things you can do to fight cancer and prepare yourself for treatment are to eat a mostly plant-based diet, maintain a healthy weight and be physically active. Although a diagnosis can be overwhelming, you have a part to play in your own treatment.
Be empowered. This is your journey!"

— Jocelyn Harrison, MPH, RD

Jocelyn Harrison is Reimagine Well's Nutrition, Exercise and Lifestyle Expert. In each chapter of Part One of this book (Diagnosis, Treatment, Healing and Wellbeing), Jocelyn will walk and talk you through this part of your journey. Right off the bat, as a patient and in your Survivorship, Jocelyn advises that you pick a few of the following on which to focus. Unless, of course, your doctor advises otherwise.

- Shoot for a balanced diet to keep your body healthy and strong. Use Choose My Plate (https://www.choosemyplate.gov/) to plan meals that include these food groups:
    - Vegetables and fruit are half of your plate
    - Lean protein - chicken, fish, beans
    - Whole grains
    - Dairy/dairy alternatives w/calcium
    - Small amounts of healthy fats- olive oil, nuts, and avocados

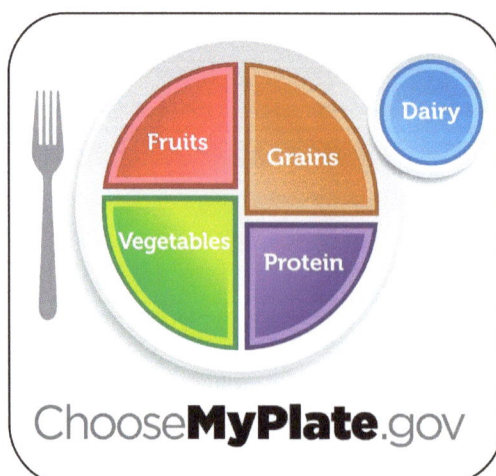

ChooseMyPlate.gov

- Make half your plate colorful vegetables, which are chock full of vitamins, minerals, fiber and phytochemicals. Phytochemicals are found naturally in plants, and are powerful cancer fighters that give plant foods their color.
- Switch out sugar sweetened beverages like sodas, sports drinks and coffee drinks for milk or water.
- Have fruit for dessert.
- If you have an exercise routine, continue it. If you don't have an exercise routine, start walking. Studies show many people with cancer feel better when they get some amount of exercise each day.
- Get your information from reliable sources. Be aware of online nutrition advice or advice from well-meaning family and friends. Healthcare professionals will provide you with the most up to date evidence-based guidance.
- Ask your doctor if there are any diet or exercise restrictions before treatment.
- Start with small changes and don't be shy about asking for help and advice.

"A Registered Dietitian (RD) is a nutrition expert. They will have the expertise and time to help you devise a nutrition plan that is both satisfying and provides your body what it needs to fight cancer."

— Jocelyn Harrison

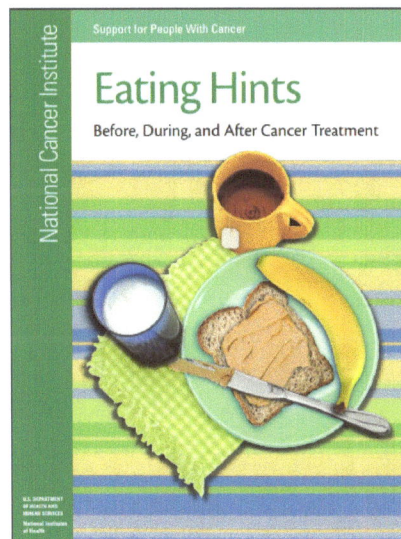

Here are some more tips that Jocelyn offers regarding any lifestyle changes a newly diagnosed cancer patient might consider.

- Take on what you can. Eating a mostly plant-based diet, daily physical activity and good sleep are the foundation of fighting cancer.
- Absolutely stop smoking if you can. Cigarette smoking damages every organ in your body and is the number one cause of death you can control. Your body will have an easier time fighting cancer without the toxic effects of cigarette smoke.

- Alcohol is also toxic to your body, and it may interfere with your medications. If you do drink, then discuss with your Care Team how alcohol might affect your treatment.
- And please, also limit the amount of processed foods like candy, cookies, pastries, sugar-sweetened beverages, and sugary coffee drinks that you consume. These foods are high in calories and low in nutrition.

TO LEARN MORE

Definition of Registered Dietitian https://www.cancer.gov/publications/dictionaries/cancer-terms?cdrid=454994

Eating Hints For Cancer Patients: https://www.cancer.gov/publications/patient-education/eating-hints

Recommendations for Cancer Prevention: http://bit.ly/2jp2DhY

Tobacco Use: http://bit.ly/2w5ZTrr

Health Goals For The Diagnosis Phase:

- Get the best Healthcare Team possible
- Find the right Hospital or Cancer Center for me
- Learn as much as possible so I can have informed and empowered discussions
- Consider "active observation" (ONLY if appropriate and decided upon in consultation with your doctor)
- Consider fertility preservation and discuss it before treatment

These are suggested goals only, please collaborate with your support community to develop your own goals for this phase.

If you are ready now to create your Bridge Plan, to help you get from Diagnosis to Wellbeing, go to: http://www.reimaginewellcommunity.com

NOTES

NOTES

Treatment

Here We Go

> "When I was diagnosed with cancer my world literally stopped. I didn't know what to do, where to go or anything. I mentally panicked…. I think most of us go into panic mode. The reason I say this is because, for most of us, after our diagnosis, we needed to gather our thoughts and make informed decisions based on viable information."
>
> — AYA Cancer Patient, Age 31, Melanoma

What Is Cancer Treatment Like?

"Cancer" is not a single disease with a one-size-fits-all approach to treatment.

If possible, it's important to be treated at a cancer hospital or a medical center which specializes in treating your type of cancer. In some cases, you should be aware that adolescents or young adults who have certain kinds of cancer may do better with treatments tailored to young children, rather than similar treatments for older adults.

As was discussed earlier, before you decide on your doctor, and a course of treatment, you should seriously consider getting a second opinion. Don't be put off by the sound of it. It's a wise thing to do. Most doctors will expect it. And you should ask if being a part of a clinical trial is also an appropriate course of treatment to consider.

Discuss all of the items in the following topics with your doctor. Bring this Learn Guide, or the hard copy of this Learn Guide, with you to each appointment. So you can be completely prepared in advance, write down, before each meeting, any questions you have for your Care Team. This will make things easier for you and for them.

TO LEARN MORE
Definition of Clinical Trial: https://www.cancer.gov/publications/dictionaries/cancer-terms?CdrID=45961

If you haven't done so already, the beginning of your treatment phase would be a great time to create and start working on your Reimagine Well Online Bridge Plan. Once you join our support community, you can interact with, learn about and get support from other cancer patients and survivors. They've been in the exact same place you are right now!

To join up, just go to:
http://www.reimaginewellcommunity.com

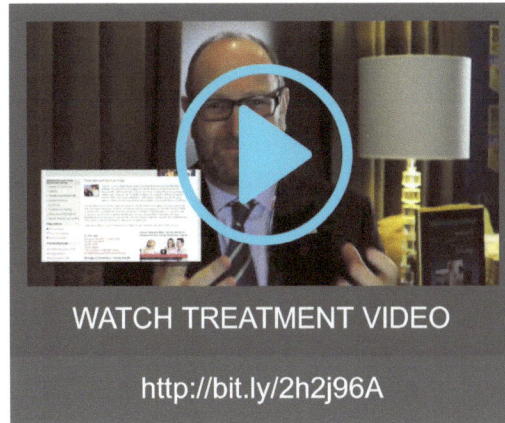

WATCH TREATMENT VIDEO

http://bit.ly/2h2j96A

The New Words You'll Be Hearing

An entire new vocabulary of words that you've never heard is about to become a part of your everyday language. The definitions of several of the key terms are below.

> "Being scared is healthy. Studying the disease helps ease the fear!"
> — AYA Cancer Patient, Age 17, Lymphoma

TUMOR. MASS. LESION.

These three words all mean the same thing: a group of abnormal cells in your body. These cells can be benign (non-cancerous) or cancerous.

PATHOLOGY.

The understanding of what your cancer looks like. To find your personal pathology, a pathologist looks at the cells under a microscope to determine the type of cancer you have.

STAGING.

This process determines if a cancer is just in the spot where it was found, or if it has moved to other body parts and organs. The staging classifications in the U.S. are the AJCC staging standards. This allows for continuity when discussing the stage of cancer across America. Staging also helps define your treatment and your prognosis.

TO LEARN MORE

Definition of Cell: https://www.cancer.gov/publications/dictionaries/cancer-terms?CdrID=46476

Definition of Benign: https://www.cancer.gov/publications/dictionaries/cancer-terms?CdrID=45614

Definition of Pathologist: https://www.cancer.gov/publications/dictionaries/cancer-terms?CdrID=46244

Definition of AJCC staging system: https://www.cancer.gov/publications/dictionaries/cancer-terms?CdrID=256554

Four Stages of Cancer:

STAGE 1

Stage 1 usually means that a cancer is relatively small and contained within the organ it started in.

STAGE 2

Stage 2 usually means the cancer has not started to spread into surrounding tissue but the tumor is larger than in stage 1. Sometimes stage 2 means that cancer cells have spread into lymph nodes close to the tumor. This depends on the particular type of cancer.

STAGE 3

Stage 3 usually means the cancer is larger. It may have started to spread into surrounding tissues and there are cancer cells in the lymph nodes in the area.

STAGE 4

Stage 4 means the cancer has spread from where it started to another body organ. This is also called secondary or metastatic cancer.

TO LEARN MORE

NCI's Adolescent and Young Adult Treatment and Clinical Trials: http://www.cancer.gov/types/aya

COG's Glossary of Cancer Terminology: https://childrensoncologygroup.org/index.php/glossary

NCI Pathology: http://www.cancer.gov/about-cancer/diagnosis-staging/diagnosis/pathology-reports-fact-sheet

NCI Staging: http://www.cancer.gov/about-cancer/diagnosis-staging/staging

If You Start With Surgery

If your doctor recommends you start your treatment with surgery, ask questions about why that decision was made. Make sure all the answers are explained clearly. Here are some important topics you should discuss in the conversations leading up to the surgery.

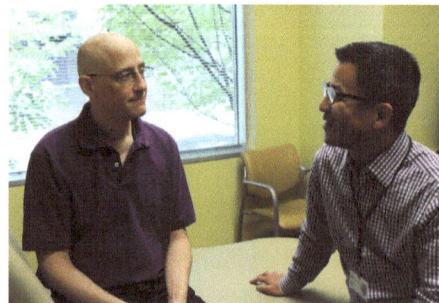

- Ask what the surgery will be like. How will it affect your body?
- It's important to talk about how you will heal after the surgery. Get the details. You should learn everything you can about the healing and recovery period.
- If you have drains in an incision site, ask how will they work. How do you take care of them? Will someone help you? Will the doctor take care of that after the surgery?

- If you have a catheter for IV medication, how do you take care of that? Remember to get the details. Ask the same questions you would ask above regarding the drains.
- Ask about pain management options. Explain your fears. Talk about if you have a high or low level of pain tolerance. Ask about the side effects of the pain medication.
- How long will you have to stay in the hospital? If you never had an overnight hospital stay, ask what that will be like. Find out if there are accommodations for family or friends to stay with you?
- What type of dressing or bandage will you have? How often should you change it?
- What changes and difference can you expect in the first day or two after the surgery?
- Will you be given instructions regarding what to eat before and after the surgery?

TO LEARN MORE
NCI's Adolescent and Young Adult Treatment and Clinical Trial: http://www.cancer.gov/types/aya

If You Start With Chemotherapy

There are over 80 types of chemotherapy (or "chemo"). Ask your doctor what kind, or kinds, you will be given. Chemotherapy may be given by mouth, injection, infusion, or on the skin. It depends on the type and stage of the cancer being treated.

Chemotherapy works by stopping or slowing the growth of cancer cells, which grow and divide quickly. But it can also harm healthy cells that divide quickly, such as those that line your mouth or intestines, or cause your hair to grow. Damage to healthy cells may cause side effects. Side effects often get better or go away after chemotherapy is over.

- Ask for a list of pros and cons to make the right decision about chemo.
- Ask about the warnings and side effects on this kind of chemo.
- Ask about how long the infusions take.
- Ask about pre- and post-chemo meds to stop the nausea and vomiting.
- How bad can the nausea and vomiting be?
- Will you lose your hair and how soon will that happen?
- What should you be eating during the chemo?
- Should you be exercising? Having sex?
- Insist you sign a consent form with all treatment information

---

TO LEARN MORE
Definition of Chemotherapy: http://bit.ly/2yorpSO
Definition of Infusion: https://www.cancer.gov/publications/dictionaries/cancer-terms?cdrid=45738
Understanding Chemotherapy: https://www.cancer.gov/publications/patient-education/understanding-chemo
Chemotherapy Basics: https://www.cancer.org/treatment/treatments-and-side-effects/treatment-types/chemotherapy.html

What Is Chemo Brain?

"Chemo Brain" refers to symptoms of fogginess of the mind, spacing out, memory lapses, or difficulty in processing or abstract reasoning. All of these may result from chemotherapy or radiation therapy. There are now new methods called 'cognitive rehabilitation' that utilize a series of tests and workshops to help rehabilitate or retrain the brain. Along with cognitive rehabilitation, it is very important to live a healthy lifestyle and be active to help stimulate your brain.

TO LEARN MORE
Chemo Brain: http://bit.ly/V4KPrB

Nutrition And Active Lifestyle During This Phase

Jocelyn Harrison, Reimagine Well's resident Registered Dietitian and Active Lifestyle Expert, has a lot of helpful information below for cancer patients. Especially those who are about to enter the treatment phase. It is extremely important that during this time you take the best care of yourself that you can, both physically and emotionally.

"Plan to have a conversation with your doctor about what to expect during treatment in terms of your diet and nutrition; also about your physical activity"

— Jocelyn Harrison

Here's a list of questions to ask your doctor before treatment:

- Are there any changes you should make to your current diet?
- Should you be taking a multivitamin? (If you are taking supplements of any kind, bring a list of what you are taking and share it with your health practitioner and dietitian.)
- If your treatment is causing you to vomit often, should you be concerned about getting necessary nutrients?
- Should you try liquid meal replacements if you have trouble keeping solid food down?
- What if you just don't feel like eating much for a couple days after treatment?

During treatment, you often have to eat foods that are different than what is considered "healthy". You will need to eat to keep your strength up and deal with the side effects of treatment. You might have a problem eating enough food, so you may need extra protein and calories. Treatment with chemotherapy and radiation is designed to kill cancer cells, but it can also harm healthy cells.

Damage to healthy cells can cause side effects that may lead to eating problems. Here are some types of eating problems that cancer treatment may cause:

- Appetite loss
- Changes in sense of taste or smell
- Constipation
- Diarrhea
- Dry mouth
- Fatigue
- Feeling full quickly
- Food aversions

- Lactose intolerance
- Nausea
- Sore mouth, tongue or throat
- Trouble swallowing
- Vomiting
- Weight gain
- Weight loss

Always talk to your doctor, nurse or dietitian about any problems on this list. There are specific steps to address each of these side effects. A dietitian can help you make changes to your diet to minimize the nutritional impact of side effects. Be wary of online nutrition advice or advice from well-meaning family and friends. Healthcare professionals will provide you with the most up-to-date evidence-based guidance.

"Studies show many people with cancer feel better when they get some exercise each day. Talk to your Care Team about an exercise plan that is right for you."

— Jocelyn Harrison

Once you've had that discussion about your exercise plan, put it into motion.

- Write out your exercise plan.
- Keep a journal about your daily progress.
- Use an online fitness app like My Fitness Pal to keep track of your physical activity and diet.
- Use a paper calendar and write down your goals or activities for the day.
- Use a fitness tracker or pedometer that tracks your steps.
- Use your Reimagine Well Patient Support Community (http://www.reimaginewellcommunity.com/) to form a group. Help each other achieve realistic health goals during treatment.

Complementary and Alternative Medicines (CAMs)

Should you consider using alternative medical therapies you may have read about, may already be practicing, or are interested in trying? These practices can include massages, relaxation exercises, vitamins, acupuncture and homeopathic medications.

They are officially referred to as complementary and alternative medicines (CAMs).

There are no studies that prove any special diet, food, vitamin, mineral, dietary supplement, herb, or combination of these can slow cancer, cure it, or keep it from coming back. As a matter of fact, some of these products can cause other problems by changing how your cancer treatment works. Your doctor can help you avoid dangerous drug-drug or drug-food interactions. If you're using a CAM now, let your doctor know.

There are some CAM approaches that have been proven to be safe and effective. Stick to the therapies that have been researched. A great place to start is the National Cancer Institute's CAM page; the link is below.

Before including any CAMs in your treatment you should always discuss them with your doctor and Care Team. Give your doctor, nurse or dietitian a list of vitamins, minerals, dietary supplements, herbs or alternative therapies you are doing, or are interested in.

"Many dietary supplements contain levels of antioxidants (such as vitamins C and E) that are much higher than the recommended Dietary Reference Intakes for optimal health. There is a concern that antioxidants might repair the damage to cancer cells that cancer treatments cause, making the treatments less effective. However, at this time the science is unclear, so it is best to avoid supplements that provide more than 100% of the Daily Value for antioxidants."

— Jocelyn Harrison

TO LEARN MORE

My Fitness Pal: https://www.myfitnesspal.com/

Definition of CAMs: https://www.cancer.gov/publications/dictionaries/cancer-terms?CdrID=44384

National Cancer Institute's CAM page: https://www.cancer.gov/about-cancer/treatment/cam

Nutrition in Cancer: http://bit.ly/2vVcQo2

Dealing With Treatment Side Effects: http://bit.ly/2f7rTrl

Dietary Reference Intakes; http://bit.ly/2wFqzic

Health Goals For The Treatment Phase:

- To make arrangements for necessary in-hospital and at home post treatment care
- To get a roadmap for the Treatment Phase of my journey
- Get informed about possible post treatment side effects and how they should be reported to my healthcare team
- Develop a diet and exercise plan that I can do while in treatment

These are suggested goals only, please collaborate with your support community to develop your own goals for this phase.

Additional Health Goals For The Treatment Phase

- Learn About Catheters and Other Important Medical Tools.
- Learn About The Sequence Of All Medical Events and Procedures.
- Learn About All The Medications You'll Be Taking.
- Learn About Diet, Exercise and Lifestyle Changes During Treatment
- Get a List Of All Medical Contacts You Might Need.

If you want to create your Bridge Plan now, to help you get from Diagnosis to Wellbeing, go to:
http://www.reimaginewellcommunity.com

NOTES

Healing

Achieving Your New Normal

"The first thing I want to say is, 'Congratulations - you are done with treatment!' Now we can concentrate on getting you to your New Normal and to adulthood. You need to understand the consequences of the therapy you've been through, and work towards wellbeing. During cancer reatment, adolescents and young adults may focus all of their energy on getting through treatment. Some may not have spent much time talking or thinking about life after cancer treatment. It's normal to have questions about returning to work or school and managing relationships. Life after treatment often presents a new set of challenges."

— Leonard Sender, M.D.

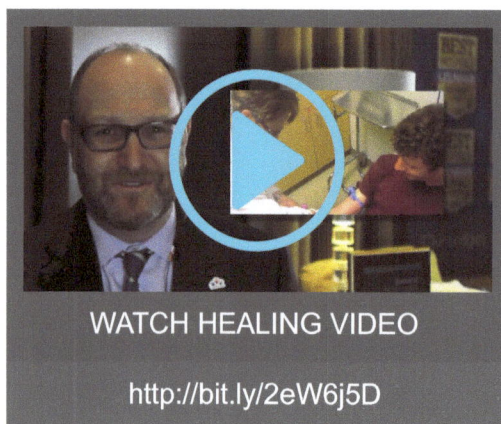

WATCH HEALING VIDEO

http://bit.ly/2eW6j5D

Before you start your Healing Phase, if you would like to join Reimagine Well's Online Support Community and create your Bridge Plan to help you get from Diagnosis to Wellbeing, Go to: http://www.reimaginewellcommunity.com.

Survivorship

While there is no exact definition of Survivorship, most agree it involves "Living with, through, and beyond cancer." In this Learn Guide, it means people in the phases after treatment, including those having no signs of cancer after finishing treatment. It also includes those who continue to have treatment over the long term, to either reduce the risk of recurrence or to manage chronic disease.

The End of Treatment Summary

At the end of your cancer treatment phase, before you move into the healing phase, you should have in your possession an End of Treatment Summary. This document should be provided to you by the medical institution where you were treated (that is your hospital or medical center), or you may compile it yourself using your own resources. An End of Treatment Summary will contain the name of your doctor and treating institution, your cancer diagnosis and the treatment you received. The Summary will include any surgeries, chemotherapy, and radiation you had. It may also list your medications, any current medical concerns, plus ongoing follow-ups and surveillance.

Every patient will have had a different cancer diagnosis and treatment. That means each individual's Summary will be different. Knowing the type of therapy you received will help you anticipate any complications that may arise because of your treatment. You can use your End of Treatment Summary as a resource to help you to communicate with your oncology team and your current primary care provider. Your current doctor should always be aware of any information about possible symptoms you may exhibit and/or future tests he or she may need to schedule in regards to your health.

You should keep your End of Treatment Summary forever. You can upload it onto an online app which contains your medical records, but we strongly recommend you keep your own paper copy. Have a backup copy, too, just for safety. If you do lose your End of Treatment Summary, you can always call the medical institution where you were treated.

TO LEARN MORE
About Survivorship: http://www.cancer.net/survivorship/about-survivorship
Follow-up Care After Cancer Treatment: https://www.cancer.gov/about-cancer/coping/survivorship/follow-up-care/follow-up-fact-sheet

Post Surgery And Post Chemo

Post surgery, post chemo - and/or post radiation - there's a new you today. And a "New Normal" to get used to! As Dr. Sender says, "Life after treatment presents a new set of challenges". Here are some things to reflect on as you begin your healing phase.

- Think about resting your body.
- Engage your body in the healing process.
- Think about and plan for the type of healthy exercise and diet you need.
- Think about and plan for sleep, meditation, and anything to have less stress.
- Heal your mind, you've been through a lot of trauma!

What Will My Follow-Up Care Be Like?

- You may have CT and PET scans to check to see if your cancer is gone.
- You may have blood tests to make sure your organs are recovering.
- You may be asked about how you are moving on with your life.
- Ask questions about managing the after-effects of surgery/chemo/radiation.
- Keep your physician apprised of any unusual symptoms you're having.

TO LEARN MORE
Definition of CT: http://bit.ly/2w6sY6m
Definition of PET: http://bit.ly/2gkdyDX

Interacting With My Care Team

As Dr. Sender states above, many things will change in your life after your treatment ends and the healing phase begins. Other aspects of your New Normal of which you should be aware are discussed in more detail below, including a whole section on nutrition and active lifestyle. Your Care Team is still there to help you, and they always will be.

Here are some issues which you should discuss with members of your Care Team, and which you need to deal with as soon as the healing phase begins:

- Allowing proper time for recovery
- Returning back to school or work
- Managing relationships with partners, family, friends and co-workers
- Returning to sexual activity/sex

A discussion right away with your primary doctor, oncologist, therapist or other members of your Care Team is recommended.

Below are some other issues which may arise during your healing phase.

Your New Normal

"We use a term called 'New Normal.' The New Normal defines for an individual what they're now capable of doing after their cancer therapy has ended. What does it mean in terms of their legs, their heart, their muscles? How do they actually maximize their potential to live a healthy, normal life for their New Normal?"

— Leonard Sender, M.D.

You'll find your New Normal by learning what your body is capable of doing. Start by revisiting everyday things you used to do. Go slow in the beginning. Take your time. See what you're feeling. Then begin to push yourself a little more every day.

- When you go for a walk, how far can you go?
- The next day, can you go a little bit farther?
- Does it hurt? What hurts? Does it continue to hurt?
- Can you run? Are you able to run a quarter of a mile? A mile?

"Cancer was just a word before 2007. It has been a rollercoaster, and it has changed who I am."
— AYA Cancer Patient, Age 30, Colorectal Cancer

Finding your New Normal doesn't happen instantly. It's a process. A process where you get in touch with your body again. It's about discovering what you're capable of doing. Now. It's about always pushing yourself just a bit out of your comfort zone. The further you get from your medical treatment, the better you're likely to feel.

Is It Normal To Be Stressed After Treatment?

"Is it normal to be stressed out after cancer treatment? Yes. Some patients have no stress, and some patients have excessive stress – it really depends on the individual. Sometimes it's just the realization that therapy has ended, and now you have time to think about what you've been through, and what you still have to go through to get to wellbeing. Please, if you are experiencing stress, talk to your healthcare professional about it – we have many ways to help."

— Leonard Sender, M.D.

Every single person has some stress after cancer treatment. That's okay. Excessive amounts of stress are bad for you, though. They don't allow healing to occur. You really need to be aware of what it means to be very stressed. Part of that awareness involves being open about, and acknowledging, the underlying reasons for that stress.

Managing Stress After Cancer Treatment

One of the ways you can manage stress is to talk about it. Talk to your family, to your friends, and your Care Team. If you're using Reimagine Well's Support Community, talk to other members to understand how they have dealt with it. Other ways to manage stress are to exercise, do meditation, practice yoga or pilates. The trick is to find activities for you that allow your body and mind to come together to heal.

TO LEARN MORE

Psychological Stress & Cancer: http://www.cancer.gov/about-cancer/coping/feelings/stress-fact-sheet
Reimagine Well Support Community: http://www.reimaginewellcommunity.com/

"Being physically active during treatment was a good thing.
It helped keep my mind clear."
— AYA Cancer Patient, Age 18, Lymphoblastic Leukemia

Low Energy After Treatment

It's normal to feel tired after a cancer treatment

Go to
http://bit.ly/2i4bwNp
to learn more about fatigue.

After cancer treatment, it's very common to have reduced energy levels. Most people do; some for quite a while. But what happens over time is they suddenly realize their energy levels have returned to normal. They're not feeling tired anymore!

There's a period of time after chemotherapy when the body is still recovering from the effects of treatment. It's normal. You'll just have to work through it.

The best way to recover from being tired is - paradoxically - to do something active. Exercise, and push your body a bit, so you RETRAIN your body. It may take three months, six months or a year before you're back, but you will come back!

TO LEARN MORE

General Info About Cancer Treatment & Fatigue: http://bit.ly/2xlrHLZ

Managing Fatigue: https://childrensoncologygroup.org/index.php/fatigue

Going Back To School And Work… And Friends

There are many challenges in going back to school and work. One of them is how you will actually do your work. For students, ask someone on your Care Team, perhaps an oncology social worker, to update your teachers. A Care Team member can help your teachers understand exactly what you're capable of doing, what therapy you've had, and what the next stages are for you.

As for work, a family member or member of your Care Team can speak to your boss or someone in Human Resources about setting fair and realistic expectations for your returning to your job.
The second part of the challenge is how you reengage with your friends. How do you make sure you get back into your social circles? How do you catch up with the life that passed by while you were in treatment? Take the time to discuss these issues, first with trusted family members, then with your very closest friends. Widen your communication circle only after you feel comfortable doing so.

Remember, you are not the first person in the world to have gone through cancer treatment. Others have experienced this before and can help you. Don't be afraid. Be proactive. Ask for help! You'll find that people are more caring and accommodating than you might expect. Asking for help goes for caregivers, too!

TO LEARN MORE

Coping After Treatment: https://www.cancer.gov/about-cancer/coping/survivorship

Coping For Caregivers: https://www.cancer.gov/about-cancer/coping/caregiver-support/caregiving-after-treatment

Children's Oncology Group: Challenges in School (https://childrensoncologygroup.org/index.php/one-year-off-treatment-and-beyond) and Learning Problems After Treatment (http://bit.ly/2fzxHXW)

Reimagine Well Support Community (http://www.reimaginewellcommunity.com/)

What Is Health Literacy?

"We think of health literacy as something that allows you to understand what therapy you've been through, what therapy meant to you – the words, the experience, the terms that describe your actual cancer – and also what it means for you in terms of getting back to wellbeing. We want you to know what it is that you need to look out for."

— Leonard Sender, M.D

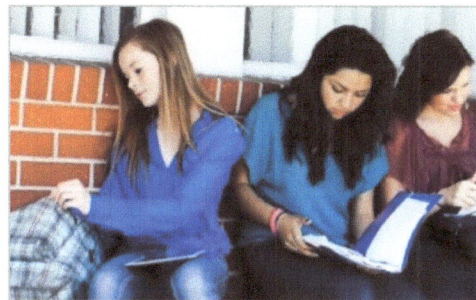

Finding Reputable Sources On The Internet

How do you know if you've gone to a credible site on the internet? Often, you don't. There are really good sites from reputable institutions like the National Cancer Institute, American Cancer Society, and the Leukemia and Lymphoma Society. Go there first to see what they have to say.

"I would tell the parents of a newly diagnosed child to be careful with the Internet. There's a lot of misconceptions out there. Information that is not true, or very dated. Listen to what the doctors tell you, and the information they give you."

— AYA Caregiver/Mom

TO LEARN MORE

Cancer Information on the Internet: http://bit.ly/2f5QrkL

Evaluating Online Sources of Health Information: http://bit.ly/2hNE252

National Cancer Institute: https://www.cancer.gov/

Children's Oncology Group: https://childrensoncologygroup.org/

American Cancer Society: http://www.cancer.org/

Leukemia and Lymphoma Society: http://www.lls.org/

Alcohol And Its Impact On Recovery

Drinking alcohol can affect recovery after cancer. Many of the chemotherapy drugs used to treat cancer in AYA patients can affect the liver's functioning. If you add alcohol into the mix, it may inhibit the liver from working properly. It may even damage it. Alcohol use after cancer really can do you some harm.

Alcohol can also interfere with post-cancer medications. It's important to discuss this with your Care Team before assuming you can go back to your old lifestyle and start drinking again. Find out from your doctors and pharmacists whether drinking alcohol may create adverse reactions with any medications you are taking.

> "Information is your friend… ask lots of question… do lots of research."
> — AYA Cancer Patient, Age 29, Leukemia

TO LEARN MORE

Straight Talk – Does Alcohol Affect My Cancer?: https://straighttalk.chocchildrens.org/young-adult-cancer/does-alcohol-affect-my-cancer/

Can Using Marijuana Affect A Teen's Recovery?

The answer is… we don't really know. One reason cancer patients use marijuana (in various ways including inhaling, ingesting, and topical applications) is because of nausea during chemotherapy. When chemotherapy is done and the nausea is over, people are often told it's not safe to use a product not yet fully understood. No one knows what the long-term implications might be for someone who's been through chemo and continues to use marijuana. Try to avoid it.

TO LEARN MORE

Definition of Inhalation: http://bit.ly/2xdSdY1

Definition of Ingestion: http://bit.ly/2w63hme

Definition of Topical: http://bit.ly/2xuVORf

Tobacco And Health

Healthcare professionals have known since the 1960's smoking tobacco cigarettes increases your risk of getting lung disease, heart disease and bladder cancers. It also impacts your breathing later in life. Smoking tobacco is never a good idea.

Will tobacco use put you at risk for future cancers? The answer is yes. Tobacco on its own increases your risk of cancer. If you've already had cancer and been through treatment that's damaged your normal tissue - and increased your risk for secondary cancer - adding tobacco massively increases your cancer risk.

As for E-cigarettes, research is being done on them right now. But nicotine in the amount found in E-cigarettes is not healthy for you. Especially if you've had chemotherapy that may have affected your liver. The long-term consequences of using electronic cigarettes is unknown. But cancer survivors shouldn't use them. They may further harm your body after it's already sustained damage from cancer.

> **Smoking tobacco INCREASES the risk of**
> - **lung disease**
> - **heart disease**
> - **bladder cancers**
>
> **and affects the ability to breathe later in life.**

TO LEARN MORE

Quitting Smoking: https://www.cancer.gov/publications/dictionaries/cancer-terms?cdrid=748251

Use of E-Cigarettes Growing Among Teens: https://blog.chocchildrens.org/use-of-cigarette-like-devices-growing-among-teens/

Taking Someone Else's Prescription Drugs

Doctors are often asked if a patient can take someone else's prescription medication. The answer is no. Every time a doctor prescribes a drug, it is prescribed to an individual person. Doctors are using their knowledge of that person's medical condition. Taking someone else's medication can not only be dangerous, it can be fatal.

TO LEARN MORE

What Parents Must Know About Prescription, OTC Drug Abuse:

https://blog.chocchildrens.org/what-parents-must-know-about-prescription-otc-drug-abuse/

How Cancer Treatment Can Affect A Young Man's Reproductive Health

Cancer treatments can destroy a young man's sperm, along with his testes. Testes function to make sperm. It is recommended that after diagnosis and before treatment, a male cancer patient do sperm banking, which saves the sperm for later use. The sperm is frozen and stored, and it may remain viable for many years.

After treatment your doctor can test to see if your sperm has returned, and if it's functioning normally. If your sperm has not returned or is not functioning normally, and you chose to do sperm banking, your doctor will remind you to keep paying the yearly fee to keep your sperm frozen until you want to use it to have a child.

Testosterone is needed for a man's sexual function. Doctors are learning about how chemotherapy can affect a male's ability to create testosterone, and therefore achieve an erection. If you are having challenges with achieving an erection you should not feel shy about discussing it with someone from your Care Team.

> "The best quality of life stands out as one of the most important issues men consider in choosing a treatment course and what to do afterward."
> — AYA Cancer Patient, Age 19, Melanoma

TO LEARN MORE

Definition of Testicle: https://www.cancer.gov/publications/dictionaries/cancer-terms?CdrID=46611

Definition of Testosterone: https://www.cancer.gov/publications/dictionaries/cancer-terms?CdrID=45581

Cancer Therapy's Effect on Male Reproductive System and Fertility Option: http://bit.ly/2x0nJ9q

Fertility Concerns and Preservation for Men: http://bit.ly/213UDxs

How Cancer Treatment Can Affect A Young Woman's Reproductive Health

If you are a young woman, cancer treatment can permanently damage your ovaries. As a result of this, your ovaries often won't be able to produce normal hormones. If the ovaries don't produce hormones, that affects your fertility. Which means there will be an inability to conceive and have children. In some cancer treatments, the ovaries are not destroyed instantly, but slowly. This means your ability to conceive and have children will lessen, and then stop over time. You will then also be likely to enter into menopause at a highly accelerated rate.

Established Options for Post-Pubertal Females

University of Colorado
Anschutz Medical Campus

- Oophoropexy
- Egg/embryo banking
- Ovarian tissue banking
- Donor eggs, adoption
- Gestational carrier

Oncofertility Program | Department of Obstetrics & Gynecology
Expanding parenthood options for life after cancer

It is often recommended that after diagnosis and before treatment, female cancer patients freeze eggs and/or embryos, or try experimental ovarian tissue transplants. This will save your eggs, embryos and ovarian tissue for later use. It requires they be frozen and stored, where it may remain viable for many years.

After your treatment is finished, your Care Team can determine whether your ovary function is normal. If your ovaries are not functioning normally, and you chose to freeze your eggs, embryos or ovarian tissue, your doctor will remind you to keep paying the fees to keep them frozen until you want to use them to have a child.

TO LEARN MORE
Definition of Ovaries: http://bit.ly/2xdboRX
Definition of Hormones: http://bit.ly/2heJtun
Effects of Children's Cancer Treatment on Female Reproductive Health:
https://childrensoncologygroup.org/index.php/hormonesandreproduction/femalereproductivehealth
Preserving Fertility in Adolescent Cancer Patients: https://blog.chocchildrens.org/preserving-fertility-adolescent-cancer-patients/

Preventing Sexually Transmitted Diseases

Just because you've had cancer and survived, it doesn't mean you can't get AIDS, gonorrhea, or syphilis. All adolescents and young adults should be concerned about sexually transmitted diseases. You should always engage in safe sex practices, be smart about your sexual activity, and use condoms.

TO LEARN MORE
How STDs Affect the AYA Population: http://www.cdc.gov/std/life-stages-populations/adolescents-youngadults.htm

Body Image After Treatment

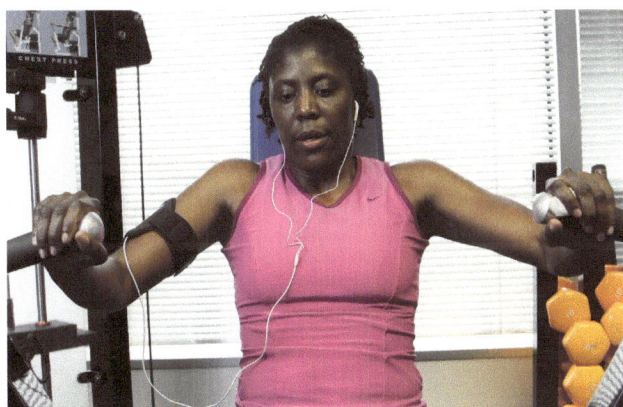

Depending on the type of treatment you received – such as surgery that includes physical scarring or an amputation, for example – there can be a huge impact on a person's body image.
Certain prescribed medications, like steroids, can promote excessive weight gain. This can also impact body image.

In the healing phase, it is important for you to seek counseling for any mental or physical issues which may be troubling you. That way your Care Team can provide coping strategies to help you adjust to your New Normal.

About 20% of cancer patients develop significant weight gain. Diet and exercise are the most important ways patients can decrease or maintain weight. This is where your BMI comes in. You'll find more information about that in the next section.

TO LEARN MORE
Definition of Amputation: http://bit.ly/2xvYfTJ
Definition of Steroids: http://bit.ly/2w5qLb2
Definition of BMI: http://bit.ly/2xlsl6e
Managing Weight After Cancer Treatment: https://www.mskcc.org/blog/8-tips-managing-weight-during-and-after-treatment
National Cancer Institute: A New Normal: http://www.cancer.gov/about-cancer/coping/survivorship/new-normal

What Does BMI Mean?

BMI is Body Mass Index. This refers to the relative amount of muscle and fat in the body as determined by your height and weight. BMI is used to determine whether you are at a healthy weight, underweight, or overweight. If you are overweight, it increases your risk for diseases such as obesity and diabetes. Being overweight can also increase the risk of a cancer recurrence.

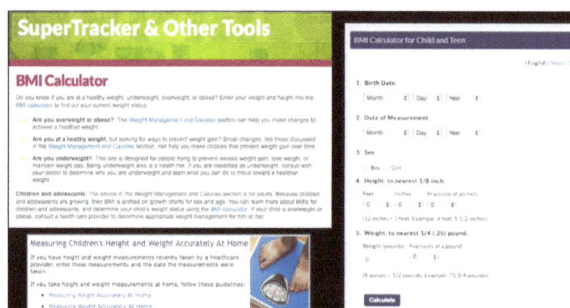

TO LEARN MORE
Calculate Your BMI: https://www.cdc.gov/healthyweight/assessing/bmi/adult_bmi/index.html
Choose My Plate SuperTracker and BMI Calculator: https://www.choosemyplate.gov/tools-supertracker

Which Foods To Avoid

There are a few fun ways to think about the foods you should avoid during your healing phase. When looking at pre-packaged food products, always check the ingredients to see if you can read and/or pronounce them. If the ingredients seem to have come out of a chemistry set, you probably shouldn't put them in your body. If there's an ingredient your great-grandmother wouldn't have recognized, think twice before you eat it.

You also really want to reduce fried foods such as French fries and potato chips. You should limit red meat, including beef, pork, and lamb. You should also limit the two S's, meaning foods high in Salt and

Sugar. Especially sugary drinks and sodas. Stick to water, instead. Or 2% milk. Or even fresh fruit juices.

As a rule, always bring the best whole foods into your kitchen. There are great recipes on www.choosemyplate.gov for teenagers, young adults and their families.

Only you can decide if you want to live a healthier, longer life. One way to look and feel better is by putting fresh, healthy, non-processed foods into your body.

TO LEARN MORE

How Food Labels Help Consumers Make Healthier Choices: http://www.fda.gov/ForConsumers/ConsumerUpdates/ucm527548.htm

Healthy Recipes from ChooseMyPlate.gov: https://www.choosemyplate.gov/recipes-cookbooks-and-menus

Feelings Of Sadness and Loneliness

After various medical procedures, particularly cancer treatment, it's normal to feel depressed or lonely. With any major change in your life, there is often a struggle to understand how that change has affected you and your family. It's also natural to have a period of grieving over the loss of time, school, friends and one's health.

> "One of the hardest things is to ask for help."
> — AYA Caregiver/Mom

At Reimagine Well, we highly recommend surrounding yourself with compassionate people who can help you understand what you've been through. Professional counselors can be contacted to be there for you during and after treatment. Close family members, friends and Care Team workers can also help work out your loneliness and sadness as you find the strength to get through your healing phase.

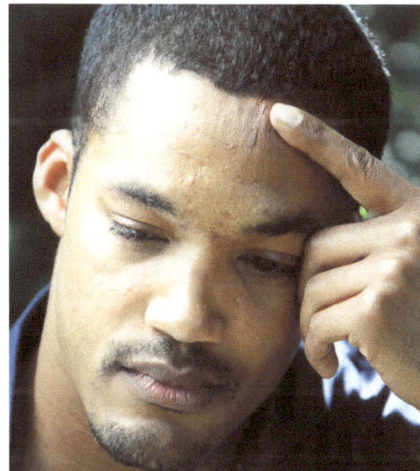

TO LEARN MORE

Definition of Grief: http://bit.ly/2f7XtBK

Get Moving And Set Exercise Goals

It's important to exercise to increase muscle and bone strength, circulation, and your focus. Exercise also increases your energy levels and helps you sleep better. Exercise every day. In the morning, if possible, to jumpstart your metabolism.

Exercise can also elevate your mood. Because when your energy levels are high, you're usually feeling your best. Meet with your doctor or a registered dietitian to set exercise goals. A good way to create exercise goals is to make them SMART:

- **S**pecific
- **M**easurable
- **A**ttainable
- **R**ealistic
- **T**imely

By setting and achieving your exercise goals, you'll move forward in finding your New Normal. To be at your best in your New Normal requires attention to diet, exercise, and emotional health. These things are important for a long, healthy life.

TO LEARN MORE
Physical Activity Tracker from ChooseMyPlate.gov: https://www.choosemyplate.gov/physical-activity

Nutrition and Active Lifestyle During This Phase

"As a result of your cancer treatment you may have lost or gained weight beyond what is healthy. One important part of cancer prevention or preventing a recurrence is to maintain a healthy weight."

— Jocelyn Harrison

After treatment, your body needs to recover. It may be some time before it's 100% of what it was. As you know, the New Normal is your optimal health after treatment. To get you to the New Normal, there are many different diets and active lifestyle choices. No one size fits all. So Reimagine Well's nutrition and lifestyle expert Jocelyn Harrison has suggestions on how to get you back on the road to wellbeing.

Goals to Reduce Future Cancer Risk

Jocelyn recommends these goals from the American Institute for Cancer Research (AICR):

- Be as lean as possible without becoming underweight.
- Be physically active at least 30 minutes a day. Moderate-intensity cardiovascular activity five times a week; muscle-strengthening exercises two days a week.
- Eat a large variety of vegetables, fruits, whole grains and legumes/beans.

- Avoid sugary drinks.
- Limit consumption of energy-dense or salty foods, particularly processed foods high in added salt, sugar and fat, and low in fiber.
- Limit consumption of red meats and avoid processed meats.
- Limit alcoholic drinks.
- Do not rely on supplements to protect you against cancer.
- Do not smoke or chew tobacco.

"Be patient with yourself and your progress. Remember: Changing behavior takes time. By making gradual changes you are much more likely to stay on track in the long run."

— Jocelyn Harrison

TO LEARN MORE

American Institute for Cancer Research (AICR): http://www.aicr.org/reduce-your-cancer-risk/recommendations-for-cancer-prevention/

Definition of Cardiovascular: (https://www.cancer.gov/publications/dictionaries/cancer-terms?CdrID=44005)

Most Important Dietary Goals

You don't have to become a vegetarian or give up the foods you love, says Jocelyn. It's your overall pattern of eating that counts.

Vegetables, fruits, whole grains and beans should always take up at least 2/3 of your plate. To maximize vitamins and minerals, choose colorful produce such as dark leafy greens, tomatoes, strawberries, blueberries, carrots and cantaloupe.

Prepare your own food. The best way to know what's in your food is to make it yourself. There are endless ways to create fresh wholesome meals. Fish, poultry, lean red meat, cheese and other animal foods should take up only 1/4 or less of your plate. Try to go meatless several times a week.

"Depending on the type and location of your cancer, your may have had surgery that alters your digestive system. For example, stomach cancer may require that part of the stomach be removed. Be sure to ask your doctor if your treatment impacts the way you can eat. Ask for a referral to a Registered Dietitian (RD) to get a healthy eating plan based on the specifics of your treatment regimen."

— Jocelyn Harrison

"When you have hope, when you have a lot of patience, cancer doesn't win!"

— AYA Caregiver/Sister

Most Important Physical Activity Goals

You don't have to join a gym or buy equipment to exercise. Physical activity can be low-cost or free. A pair of supportive rubber-soled shoes and a Youtube video can start you on your way. Any sidewalk can be an Olympic running track.

Break up your 30 minutes of daily activity into 10-to-15 minute sessions. This provides the same health benefits. If you sit a lot, take walks every two hours.

If you resolve to exercise for 30 minutes a day and then miss a day, don't give up. Forgive yourself and get back to it! Try a different time of day if that works for you.

Use physical activity as your personal "me" time. Or you may get more motivated by joining a class or having an activity buddy. Either way... exercise!

Specific Goals Are The Best Goals!

- Focus on individual goals. Don't make huge, drastic changes overnight.
- Ask for help. Find a registered dietitian (RD) and a certified exercise physiologist.
- Go public with your health goals. Set a specific goal. Tell others about it.

- Record your behavior. Track your progress or change your goal if you need to.
- Reward yourself. When you reach milestones along the way to your goal.
- Accept setbacks. Deal with setbacks, work through them, then get back on track!

You're Taking All My Fun Away!

Living a healthy lifestyle can be fun! It can have a dramatic, positive effect on how you feel. It all sounds overwhelming at first, but hang in there. Start by collecting healthy recipes that you love. Luckily, we live in a time of bountiful fresh produce and endless ways to prepare it. If you need to have fun, follow the 90/10 rule. Do what's best for your health 90% of the time. You can still enjoy your treats. But make them the exception.

I Don't Feel Supported By My Family And Friends

Sometimes our friends, and even our family members, don't seem to be able to support us with our diet and lifestyle changes. If that's the case for you, Jocelyn suggests it might be helpful to find a local cancer support group in your community. Sit in on a few sessions and join it if you're comfortable. That way you can connect with others who are on a similar cancer journey. Your doctor, social worker or dietitian may be able to help.

TO LEARN MORE

Nutrition And Staying Active During/After Cancer Treatment: http://bit.ly/2mYINZR

Nutrition After Treatment Ends: http://bit.ly/2s5iMJ6

Reimagine Well's Online Support Community: http://www.reimaginewellcommunity.com/reimaginewell

And don't forget Reimagine Well's Online Support Community!

Health Goals For The Healing Phase:

- Plan ahead for any school or work issues - allow time
- Speak to my doctor about any issues in being sexually active
- Develop a healthy diet (whole organic foods, less animal protein, with greens and fresh fruit)
- Create an appropriate exercise program
- Develop more goals on your own

(These are suggested goals only, please collaborate with your support community to develop your own goals for this phase.)

If you are ready to create your Bridge Plan, to help you get from Diagnosis to Wellbeing, go to: http://www.reimaginewellcommunity.com

NOTES

Wellbeing

It's Your Future

"Going forward, it's important to have follow-up care visits, which can help prevent or detect any problems due to cancer or its treatment. Follow-up care can help assure that emotional issues and concerns are addressed. Talk with your doctor to learn more. Learn how others have gotten back to living their lives!"

— Leonard Sender, M.D.

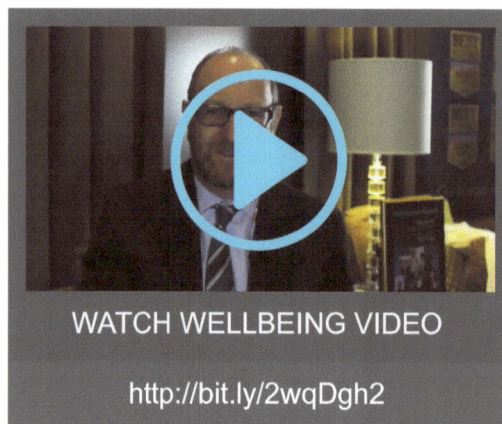

WATCH WELLBEING VIDEO

http://bit.ly/2wqDgh2

You've probably already joined the Reimagine Well's Online Support Community, but if you haven't, you're missing out on something that many AYA survivors have found to be very helpful. Cancer survivors like you are there, asking and answering questions, posting blogs and Tips 4 Life. Maybe you're a private person, or maybe you just haven't had the time to create your Bridge Plan. Find the time. Go to: http://www.reimaginewellcommunity.com

Wellbeing - How Do I Face My Future?

It's all about looking at your body and thinking about PREVENTION! Dr. Sender believes the single most important thing you can do to prevent recurrence of cancer is to maintain a healthy body weight by eating a balanced diet and exercising regularly. Or in one easy sentence: focus on healthy living and set goals to keep you healthy.

- Make a detailed recording, or create written notes, of what your treatment was. Keep a copy of your End Of Treatment Summary handy. That way you can talk to other doctors in detail about it if you need to. It is crucial for other doctors to be able to understand what you had done.
- Depending on the type of cancer you had, you may need occasional re-scans and blood tests. That's to make sure the cancer is gone for up to five years after your last treatment.
- Live with and beyond your cancer. If you take care of yourself and be smart, your New Normal can be more fulfilling than ever before!
- Give back to other AYAs. Do this by sharing lessons you've learned in places like the Reimagine Well Support Community (http://www.reimaginewellcommunity.com/). In that private, online platform you can help the other adolescents and young adults following in your footsteps.

- Consider participating in post-treatment studies though your hospital or with your doctor.
- Finally, keep using and working on your Bridge Plan. Communicate with the people you've met in your community. Exchange ideas and suggestions. Set new achievable health goals every year.

Is Wellbeing A State of Mind?

"Absolutely! Wellbeing is really how you think of yourself in the context of your life. What your spiritual life is like, what your physical life is like, what your emotional life is like. Gather a lot of friends around you. Give back to society. Find meaningful employment, find meaning in your life."

— Leonard Sender, M.D.

The First Five Years

The first five years after your cancer treatment ends are very important. The chances your cancer will return are highest in the first two years. The farther away you are from the end of treatment, the smaller the chances your cancer will come back. That is why doctors set a five year goal in your cancer journey.

Follow Up During The First Five Years

The follow-up for the first five years will depend on your cancer diagnosis. You will normally be seen by your doctor at frequent intervals in the first few years, and then ongoing check-ups will gradually be spaced apart. There may be recommendations for blood tests and imaging studies, depending on your diagnosis and treatment. During this time your Care Team should also ensure that you're recovering from all possible complications which may have occurred during your treatment.

TO LEARN MORE

What is follow-up cancer care, and why is it important?:

https://www.cancer.gov/about-cancer/coping/survivorship/follow-up-care/follow-up-fact-sheet#q1

What should patients tell their doctor during follow-up visits?:

https://www.cancer.gov/about-cancer/coping/survivorship/follow-up-care/follow-up-fact-sheet#q2

How are follow-up care schedules planned?:

https://www.cancer.gov/about-cancer/coping/survivorship/follow-up-care/follow-up-fact-sheet#q3

Are there doctors or clinics that specialize in follow-up care?:

https://www.cancer.gov/about-cancer/coping/survivorship/follow-up-care/follow-up-fact-sheet#q4

What should patients talk to their doctor about once cancer treatment ends?:

https://www.cancer.gov/about-cancer/coping/survivorship/follow-up-care/follow-up-fact-sheet#q5

How can patients deal with their emotions once cancer treatment is completed?:

https://www.cancer.gov/about-cancer/coping/survivorship/follow-up-care/follow-up-fact-sheet#q6

What kinds of medical information should patients keep?:

https://www.cancer.gov/about-cancer/coping/survivorship/follow-up-care/follow-up-fact-sheet#q7

What other services may be useful during follow-up care?:

https://www.cancer.gov/about-cancer/coping/survivorship/follow-up-care/follow-up-fact-sheet#q8

What research is being done in regards to follow-up cancer care?:

https://www.cancer.gov/about-cancer/coping/survivorship/follow-up-care/follow-up-fact-sheet#q9

Does NCI have guidelines for follow-up care?:

https://www.cancer.gov/about-cancer/coping/survivorship/follow-up-care/follow-up-fact-sheet#q10

"The most important thing that I would say… after the 5 year mark is to be encouraged and keep going! Share your story! You can help other people, and this is how we learn from each other. All of your knowledge becomes our knowledge – this is how we encourage and empower one another."

— Lilibeth Torno, M.D.

TO LEARN MORE

National Cancer Institute: Follow-up Care After Cancer Treatment: http://bit.ly/2y7awMc

ASCO Cancer Treatment Summaries and Survivorship Care Plans: http://bit.ly/1Hd7O9k

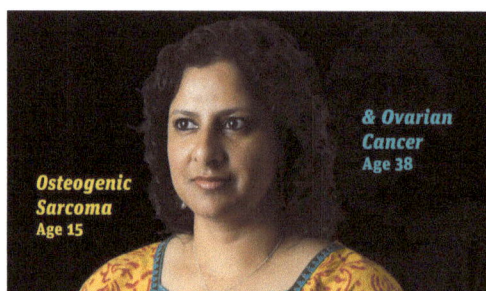

Working Toward Independence

Whether you are an AYA cancer survivor in your teens, 20's or 30's, after your healing phase, the time will come when you'll have to take charge of your own life. When your parents and/or caregivers will return to their regular routines and obligations. That's when you'll find your new way of living as an independent person.

Jenee Areeckal, pediatric and AYA oncology social worker - and a three-time AYA cancer survivor herself - has some suggestions for your journey:

"The things I hope you would pay more attention to would be your emotional wellbeing, physical wellbeing, and your follow-up care. For long-term Survivorship, you need to get The End of Treatment Summary - a folder describing your diagnosis, your treatment, and side effects of your therapy. What I recommend young adults do is to give a copy of that document to their primary care doctor, at home, on the road, or in college. The person who is most responsible for your Survivorship is YOU. You need to be the advocate and the leader in your own care."

Staying In Touch

Social workers, nurses, child-life specialists and doctors love to hear from you. They've shared a journey with you, so your updates only help them to see how far you've come, and your successes. For them, that brings immense satisfaction and gratitude.

"Prior to cancer, being an athlete was my passion. When I was diagnosed with osteosarcoma and lost my leg, I never thought I could still do sports. I took a beginning class thinking I couldn't swim. When I got into the pool, I realized I could – it was just a matter of learning a new way of swimming, just like I learned how to play tennis in a wheelchair. I thought I needed two legs to ski, but found out that I didn't - I am called a 3-track skier. It turns out I could be, can be, and am an athlete again! This is my 'new' athletic way of playing."

— Jenee Areeckal

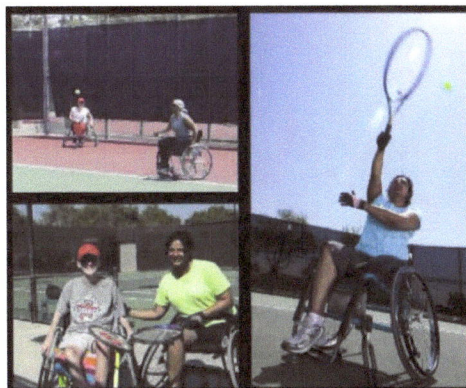

Resources To Help You Find Your New Way of Living

> "The return to "normal,"
> though gradual and not complete,
> has been wonderful."
> — AYA Cancer Patient, Age 25, Liver Cancer

Jenee recommends that as you adjust to your new way of living, it's good to use outside resources for advice. They are easily accessible and happy to help you connect with other cancer survivors who have gone through similar situations as you. Try organizations such as SeventyK.org, STUPIDCANCER, American Cancer Society, NCI AYA Page and our own Reimagine Well Support Community (http://www.reimaginewellcommunity.com/).

"A way to move past cancer is by using something you're passionate about," Jenee told Reimagine Well, "In my case it was being an athlete. I connected with the Challenged Athletes Foundation. They were able to help me get active again. For you, it might be something like trying to write about your story." She recommends finding an organization or a resource that can help develop your passion!

> **Resources to help you find your 'New Normal':**
> - **Your social worker**
> - **A psychologist**
> - **Your doctors**
> - **Family members**
> - **Outside organizations in the cancer world**

TO LEARN MORE

Resources for Teen Cancer Survivors: http://www.cancer.net/navigating-cancer-care/teens/resources-teens

ACS Cancer Survivors Network: http://csn.cancer.org/

SeventyK.org

Stupid Cancer: http://stupidcancer.org/connect/

American Cancer Society: https://www.cancer.org/content/cancer/en_header.html

NCI AYA Page: https://www.cancer.gov/types/aya

Challenged Athletes Foundation: http://www.challengedathletes.org/

An Active Lifestyle Means A Healthy Lifestyle

As you've already learned, nutrition and exercise play a huge role in your long-term goals of wellbeing. A lot of things have happened to your body – different kinds of treatment, medications, chemotherapy, surgery. After going through that, you really want to make sure your body is healthy. So give it a good diet and… exercise!

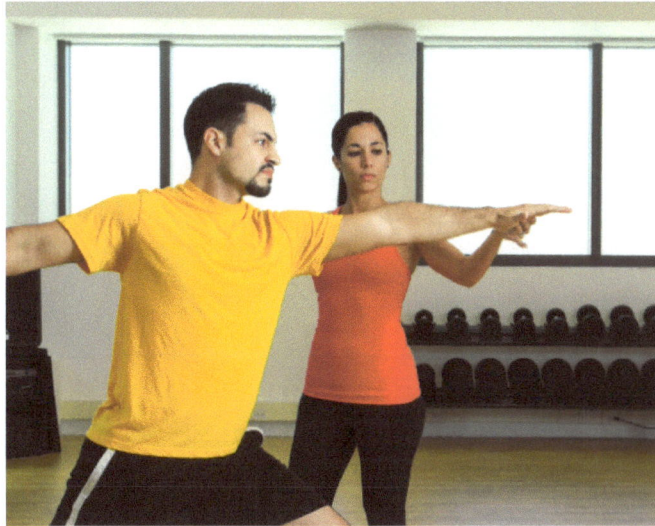

TO LEARN MORE

Staying Healthy Through Diet and Physical Activity: http://www.survivorshipguidelines.org/pdf/DietandPhysicalactivity.pdf

Guidelines for a Healthy Lifestyle: https://www.cancer.gov/about-cancer/coping/survivorship/follow-up-care

Being Healthy After Treatment Ends: http://www.cancer.org/treatment/survivorshipduringandaftertreatment/behealthyaftertreatment/index

Setting Long-Term Health Goals

The very first long-term health goal you should set is keeping your body healthy. In addition to Dr. Sender's advice about a good diet and lots of exercise, a healthy body also includes exercising your brain, your mind and your soul. Those are all great goals to set and keep long-term. Included in your goals should also be career plans, making friends and exploring relationships.

You need to get back into society. Get back to living. Start by making simple, SMART goals. That will set you up to be a GREAT survivor!

> "My goal is to become a Pediatric Oncology Nurse within the next few years!"
> — AYA Cancer Patient, Age 25, Leukemia

TO LEARN MORE

Healthy Living Guidelines for Cancer Survivors: http://bit.ly/2fjYnMj

Nutrition and Lifestyle in Cancer Survivors: http://bit.ly/2y6zcEx

Getting a Wellness Plan: https://www.cancer.gov/about-cancer/coping/survivorship/follow-up-care

SMART Goals: https://www.reimaginewellcommunity.com/node/7623

Long-term goals:

- **Follow a healthy diet**
- **Exercise regularly**
- **Stimulate the mind**
- **Take care of the soul**
- **Look into different career paths**
- **Spend time with friends**
- **Get back into LIVING!**

Get Busy Living!

"What I mean by 'get busy living' is that I love to lead a healthy, active lifestyle. Get back into society. Be a part of your community. Do sports and have fun, like any other young adult would. Get back to your friends, get back into playing and being the fun person that you are. The world may look different, but you're still you."

— Jenee Areeckal

A Final Thought From Jenee

Just remember one thing…

You're a Survivor!

Nutrition/Active Lifestyle

Near the end of this Learn Guide's previous chapter there's a section called Nutrition and Active Lifestyle. Diet and exercise is also very important during your wellbeing phase, so we would like to suggest that you revisit this section of the Learn Guide. It is in (Section C: Healing - A "New Normal").

Being A Mentor

Moving forward, you may feel you would like to mentor others. Would you like to share your experiences with another cancer patient? Often this is a patient who is experiencing what you have already gone through. By doing this, you empower them. You give them hope. And you strengthen them for what lies ahead. You can mentor other patients by volunteering at the hospital where you were treated, or your own local hospital. You can help in an online community or by phone. To do so, contact one of the services below.

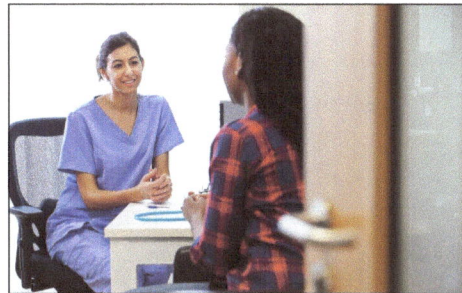

Getting Mentored

You may also feel as if you need a mentor. Someone to help you move forward into your Survivorship. There are many places where you can find someone to talk to, and perhaps even spend some time with. These services do exist. As the expression goes: help is just a phone call away. You'll find a list of links to these services below.

TO LEARN MORE

4th Angel – Patient & Caregiver Mentoring Program: http://www.4thangel.org/

Cancer Connects Volunteer Mentor Program: http://www.cancerconnects.org/volunteerMentorProgram

Imerman Angels: http://imermanangels.org/

Our Online Support Community

As you leave the wellbeing phase and head into your Survivorship, we again want to suggest you visit our Reimagine Well Support Community. It's a place where patients, survivors, caregivers and healthcare professionals share their knowledge.

"Using the support community… gives me the opportunity to know that I'm not alone, that there are others experiencing it real-time, and from whom I can learn something and contribute to them in return. And it's PRIVATE! Like, not out there on my social network..."

— AYA Cancer Patient, Age 19, Uterine Cancer

**To reach the Reimagine Well Support Community,
go to http://www.reimaginewellcommunity.com/reimaginewell.**

Health Goals For The Wellbeing Phase:

- Develop a healthy "anti-cancer" diet (whole organic foods, less animal protein, with greens and fresh fruit)
- Develop and maintain a proper exercise program
- Consider giving back to AYA patients following in your footsteps
- Consider participation in post treatment studies
- Develop more goals on your own

These are suggested goals only, please collaborate with your support community to develop your own goals for this phase.

NOTES

NOTES

Thoughts About Your Cancer Returning

During and after your wellbeing phase, you will wonder about this: "What if my cancer comes back?" It's part of your New Normal. So be aware of a few things. It may help ease your mind.

- It is important to keep your scheduled check-ups. This is so your doctor will be able to detect any further complications that may happen in the future.
- Your doctors will also want to make sure you are recovering well from past complications that you may have undergone.
- If you move or go out of state, make sure you comply with your doctor's recommendations for your follow-up visits.
- Participate in post-treatment studies. You can help not only yourself but others.

"Stay on the positive. Don't think about what if. Take every day for what it's worth. Don't worry about what tomorrow's going to bring, or what happened yesterday. Just focus on this day and make the best of it!"

— AYA Cancer Caregiver/Mom

What Are My Chances Of Cancer Recurrence?

Recurrence is when your cancer comes back. The chances of recurrence in the first five years will depend on your cancer diagnosis. However, we know that the chances of recurrence are highest in the two years after you stop treatment. It is important to find any recurrence of cancer early so your doctor can treat the disease appropriately before it causes more damage to your body.

At the end of five years, the chances of recurrence will be much smaller. The farther away you get from the end of your treatment, the lower the chances your cancer will come back.

TO LEARN MORE

Children's Oncology Group: Relapse or Recurrence: https://childrensoncologygroup.org/index.php/relapse

Remain Vigilant For Symptoms of Recurrence

It's important for you to remember the original symptoms that you had. Whether it was headaches, fever, fatigue, or a lump in the body. Any changes you experience have to be reported to your doctor. Immediately. The MOST IMPORTANT thing is that if you feel different or notice something out of the ordinary, you need to see your doctor right away.

Signs Your Cancer May Have Returned

Cancer recurrence will depend on the type of cancer you had originally. Each type of cancer has its own name, treatment, and prognosis (chance of responding to treatment). Cancer in Children can be divided into three groups:

- Leukemias: cancers of the blood-forming cells
- Lymphomas: cancers of the lymphatic system
- Solid tumors: cancers of the bone, muscle, brain, organs, or other tissues in the body.

If you had a SOLID TUMOR type of cancer, you may have a lump, or this may be picked up by a scan.

"When I had my recurrence, my oncologist wanted to keep me as positive as possible, as that would help me fight the hardest."
— AYA Cancer Patient, Age 30, Non-Hodgkin's Lymphoma

If you had a SKIN CANCER, you may notice the reappearance of moles, or other spots on your body. Or you may just not feel right.

Although melanoma is still rare in adolescents and young adults, you should make checking for moles part of your monthly routine.

Look for the ABCDs of moles:

- **A**symmetry
- **B**order
- **C**olor
- **D**iameter.

"Get to know your skin. If all the moles look the same and one is different, that's the one you need to worry about," Dr. Sender says. "It should never be bigger than a pencil eraser."

Where Your Cancer Can Return

Doctors define recurrent cancers by where they develop. The different types are:

- Local Recurrence. This means the cancer is in the same place as the original cancer, or is very close to it.
- Regional Recurrence. This is when the tumors grow in lymph nodes or tissues near the place of the original cancer.
- Distant Recurrence. In these cases, the cancer has spread (metastasized) to organs or tissues far from the place of the original cancer.

Local cancer may be easier to treat than regional or distant cancer. But this can be different for each patient. Talk with your doctor about options.

If It Does Return, What Do I Do Now?

If there is a recurrence of cancer, there is usually always a treatment plan that can be formulated. It is best to immediately reconnect with your cancer specialist. That way the treatment team can come up with the plan that is appropriate for your specific cancer. There is a now tremendous amount of cancer research going on in the United States and across the world. This research continues to lead to scientific breakthroughs that will translate into new treatment options for many cancer patients. In the meantime:

- Find the right hospital or clinic, and the right doctor.
- Get the best drugs and the best thinking available.

TO LEARN MORE

National Cancer Institute: When Cancer Returns: https://www.cancer.gov/publications/patient-education/when-cancer-returns.pdf

Hyundai Hope On Wheels Biorepository: https://www.childrensoncologygroup.org/index.php/hyundai-hope-on-wheels-biorepository

What Is Secondary Cancer?

A secondary cancer is a distinct cancer, separate from your original primary cancer. Depending on the type of treatment received - and also depending on genetic predisposition - some people may be more at risk for secondary cancer

TO LEARN MORE

Understanding Your Risk of Developing Secondary Cancer:

https://www.nccn.org/patients/resources/life_after_cancer/understanding.aspx

Health Link: Reducing the Risk for Second Cancers: http://bit.ly/2fjA0hy

Long Term Effects Of My Cancer Treatment

Long-term effects of cancer treatment may take many years to manifest. So it's important for you to remain watchful just in case they occur.

TO LEARN MORE

National Cancer Institute: Survivorship: https://www.cancer.gov/about-cancer/coping/survivorship

Children's Oncology Group: Late Effects of Treatment: http://bit.ly/2fjKP3n

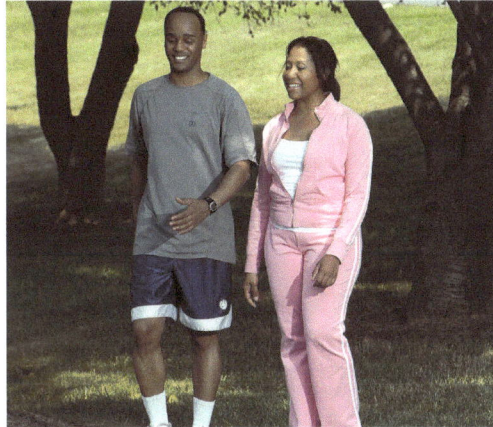

"Keep healthy. Keep your spirits up.
Live every day to the fullest. Research new procedures!!!"

— AYA Cancer Patient, Age 28, Breast Cancer

What Are Genomics

Genomics is a growing area of medical study that uses knowledge about genetic makeup, discovered through DNA sequencing, to help make medical decisions.

DNA sequencing of a person's normal cells is used to study the genes inherited from one's parents to see if the cause of a cancer may have been present since birth. This is called a hereditary mutation. Knowledge of a hereditary gene mutation can help predict future cancer risks for an individual and potentially, that individual's family members. Over 10% of pediatric cancers have a hereditary cause. Consequently, there may be risks to other family members of that patient and their future offspring. Knowing these possibilities in advance could lead to better care for the whole family.

DNA testing of the cancer cell itself is also important. DNA sequencing will show the mutations in an individual's cancer cell; a cancer cell always has mutations, mostly acquired, occasionally hereditary. This information can play a large part in an individual's clinical cancer care and treatment - knowing the genetic makeup of a cancer can guide treatment choices. It may also predict which treatments the cancer will respond to. Ask your doctor if hereditary and/or cancer DNA sequencing is useful for your cancer.

TO LEARN MORE

Definition of DNA Sequencing: https://www.cancer.gov/publications/dictionaries/cancer-terms?cdrid=753867

Definition of Genetic Profile: https://www.cancer.gov/publications/dictionaries/cancer-terms?cdrid=561400

Definition of Hereditary: http://bit.ly/2fi2yLy

What Are Genomics?: https://www.cancer.gov/publications/dictionaries/cancer-terms?cdrid=446543

Understanding Genetic Testing for Cancer: http://bit.ly/2fjjmPa

How genes can help in the diagnosis and treatment of cancer: http://bit.ly/2vUGcD8

DNA Sequencing: https://www.cancer.gov/publications/dictionaries/cancer-terms?cdrid=753867

What Is Targeted Therapy?

Targeted therapy is a newer type of cancer treatment that uses drugs or other substances to more precisely identify and attack cancer cells. Targeted therapy is a growing part of the treatment for many types of cancer.

TO LEARN MORE

What Is Targeted Therapy?: https://www.cancer.gov/publications/dictionaries/cancer-terms?cdrid=270742

How does targeted cancer therapy work?:

https://www.cancer.org/treatment/treatments-and-side-effects/treatment-types/targeted-therapy/what-is.html

What Is Immunotherapy?

Immunotherapy is another new cancer treatment that helps the body's immune system to kill cancer cells.

TO LEARN MORE

What Is Immunotherapy?: https://www.cancer.gov/publications/dictionaries/cancer-terms?cdrid=45729

What is cancer immunotherapy?: http://bit.ly/2n9H4il

What Are Clinical Trials?

Clinical trials are important for discovering what types of new treatments work. This information is impossible to gather without patients willing to participate in clinical trials. All the advances we now have come from results discovered this way. No drug in the United States is available without going through three rounds of controlled clinical trials.

Clinical trials are an important option for cancer patients since they provide the most up-to-date treatments. Currently, only about two percent of patients 20 to 39 years old are treated in clinical trials.

Participation of more adolescents and young adults in these trials will improve treatment, survival, and understanding of cancers in patients through this age group.

TO LEARN MORE
NCI Clinical Trials: http://www.cancer.gov/about-cancer/treatment/clinical-trials
What Is a Clinical Trial?: https://childrensoncologygroup.org/index.php/what-is-a-clinical-trial

A Serious Talk

In some cases, when your cancer does return, and it is severe and life-threatening, there are certain serious talks to be held with your doctors and other Care Team members.

Depending on the diagnosis, there may be a discussion about palliative or comfort care.

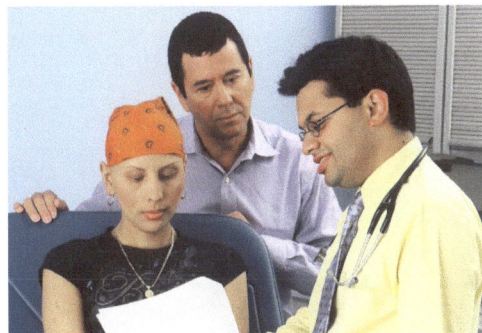

Palliative Or Comfort Care

Many people who have cancer, or who have been treated for cancer, develop symptoms or side effects that affect their quality of life. Care given to help patients cope with these symptoms or side effects is called palliative care, comfort care, supportive care, or symptom management.

Closing Words From Dr. Sender

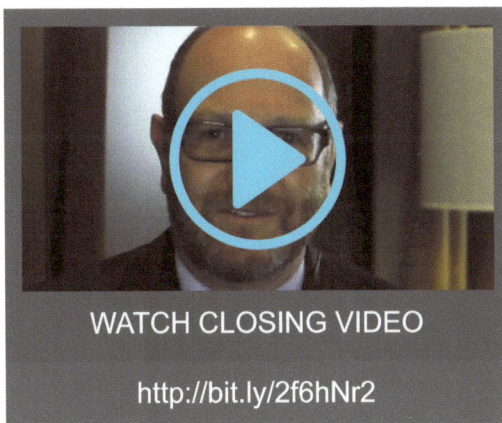

WATCH CLOSING VIDEO

http://bit.ly/2f6hNr2

"The most important thing I can say to you as an AYA cancer patient is to be positive. Every patient is unique. Surround yourself with your friends, and be positive. There is a lot of great research going on with more and more survivors every day."
— Leonard Sender, M.D.

"If you, or somebody you care about, has been diagnosed with cancer, we're here to help you get from diagnosis to wellbeing."

— Team Reimagine Well

In Part One of this Learn Guide, our goal was to supply you with informational and educational material, give you important questions to ask your doctors, and the support you needed to become an empowered patient. We did that because an empowered patient is able to actively participate in their ongoing healthcare decisions.

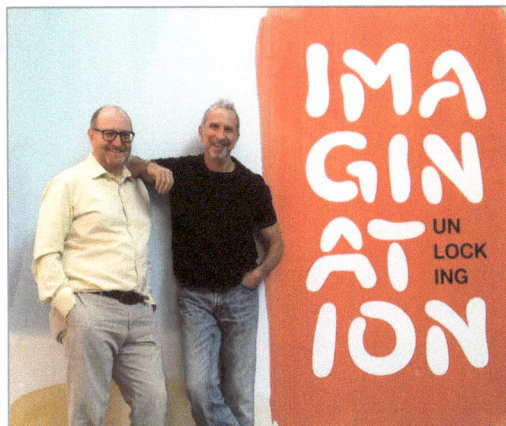

In Part Two of the Learn Guide, Reimagine Well will provide you with a safe, private place to gather your community, then use their strength, wisdom and support as you move through your journey toward Survivorship. Our patient and family community platform also aspires to guide you in setting achievable health goals at each phase of your journey. All of the blogs and tips for life you'll find here have been reviewed by our medical staff and/or the National Cancer Institute prior to being published.

This step-by-step guide will help you get started on your Reimagine Well Bridge Plan (http://www.reimaginewellcommunity.com/reimaginewell): your health plan for life. Keep it on your phone or tablet. Print it out as a chronical of your cancer journey. If you need assistance at any point along the way, you can contact a member of our staff via the "Connect" link on our website at www.ReimagineWell.com.

Yours In Health,
Leonard Sender, M.D. and Roger Holzberg - Co-Founders

Survival UP!

"Surround yourself with your friends, and be positive."

— Leonard Sender, M.D.

From Diagnosis to Treatment, Healing and Wellbeing

We promised you at the start you would not be alone.

You're not. We're here.

And so are many, many others. Especially the healthcare professionals, other cancer patients and devoted caregivers who have been here before you.

"You have to become empowered to ask the right questions. And to find the right questions, to get the information you need… we want for you to become fully engaged in the process."

— Leonard Sender, M.D.

"When you're in the heat of battle… remember why you're fighting!"

— AYA Caregiver/Mom

"I knew I needed to hear what my doctors were saying, but just as important to me was what others, just like me, did to get through the minefield… Empower yourself!"

— Roger Holzberg, Co-Founder and Cancer Survivor

"I gathered my strong friends… my greatest allies… and I made my plan… the most important thing is to figure out your battle plan."

— AYA Cancer Patient, Age 18, Germ Cell Tumors

"The world may look different, but you're still you."

— Jenee Areeckal, MSW, LCSW

"Keep being strong and spreading the message."

— AYA Cancer Patient, Age 27, Sarcoma

"By making gradual changes you are much more likely to stay on track in the long run."

— Jocelyn Harrison, MPH, RN

"Glad to see you on this site. Looking forward to helping each other."

— AYA Cancer Patient, Age 31, Cervical Cancer

Getting Started On Your Bridge Plan

The Reimagine Well Community™ is a private online and offline (printed book) guided support network that helps patients transition from diagnosis to wellbeing. Reimagine Well's patient and caregiver support community is a safe place for patients, families and staff to:

- Offer support to one another.
- Set achievable health goals in each phase of their cancer journey.
- Share best-practices for others following in their footsteps.
- Print their guide as a chronicle of the journey from diagnosis to wellbeing.

It eases the overwhelming nature of a life-threatening diagnosis by dividing the journey into manageable phases. It assists with setting achievable health goals in each phase for patients, their caregivers, supporters, community, and healthcare professionals. And it builds a health plan for life in the process.

Our support community also enables healthcare professionals to continue guidance post-treatment, through the healing and wellbeing phases of the journey.

> "This is an amazing tool and resource for newly diagnosed patients and their families. I know that my journey would have been so much different if I'd had this support when I was just starting out."
> — AYA Cancer Survivor, Age 23, Colon Cancer

Creating Your Bridge Plan

> To become a part of the Reimagine Well Support Community go to
> http://www.reimaginewellcommunity.com/

If you're just getting started, once you're registered, the first things we can do is to reduce your sense of isolation by helping you build your support community.

The next few pages are the technical stuff. (All of it is contained in the Help section of the Support Platform, too.) If you have ever made a Facebook, Instagram, YouTube, Twitter or other social media account, you'll fly right through this part!

Fill In The Personal Information

You'll be asked for the following information. Make sure it's all handy.

- Name
- Username
- Email (plus confirm email)
- Password (plus confirm password - you'll choose your own)
- Date Of Birth
- What Your Role Is (Patient or Caregiver)
- Location
- Illness
- Stage
- Enter The Confirmed Code

Registration Is Complete

As soon as you register and hit "Submit," you will be taken to your Bridge Plan. A yellow box there will include a few tips on how to start the Bridge Plan. Once you leave this page, the yellow box will disappear. Don't worry, as you will receive an email containing the same information. If you don't see the email in your inbox, check your spam folder.

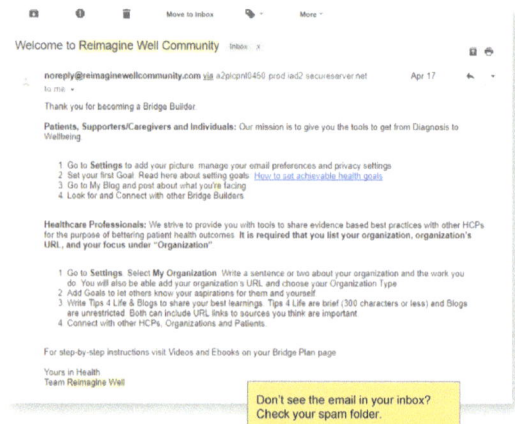

To Personalize Your Plan

To personalize your Bridge Plan, click on Settings in the top navigation box. If you provide further information to your Bridge Plan, that will allow easier access to the people, resources and data that is relevant to you.

Some of those questions will include whether you are a patient (that is anyone who has received a cancer diagnosis); a Caregiver or Supporter (which includes any family members or friends who support patients); Individuals (which is anyone interested in a building a Bridge Plan and using the resources of the website); and Healthcare Professionals (who are those in the healthcare field.)

There are also tabs here for Privacy Settings, which allows you to decide which information you want to share with other Bridge Builders; and A Description Of Your Illness, where you may describe the type of cancer for which you are being treated, or that of the patient you are supporting. You MUST always save your changes.

You must **SAVE** changes.

"The Reimagine Well support network helped me pull together my team, my strongest allies, and then helped me create my battle plan."

— AYA Cancer Patient, Age 35, Prostate Cancer

Passwords and Settings

Regarding your username. If you are not comfortable using your real name, you may select a fictional or pen name.

Passwords. Everyone has a million of them. You should write down your Password and Username in a safe place in case you forget it. If you need to change your original password, you may do that here at Settings.

Your email address will be kept private and not shared with anyone else. We will only use it to contact you.

You must **SUBMIT** changes.

If you add or change something in Settings, hit the Submit button to save those changes. Always remember to Save Your Changes.

Picture or Photograph

You may add a picture or photo on the Settings page. A photo is a good way to personalize your Bridge Plan. As with your Username, it can be an "avatar" photo if you aren't comfortable with using your own image. Then SAVE the added photo.

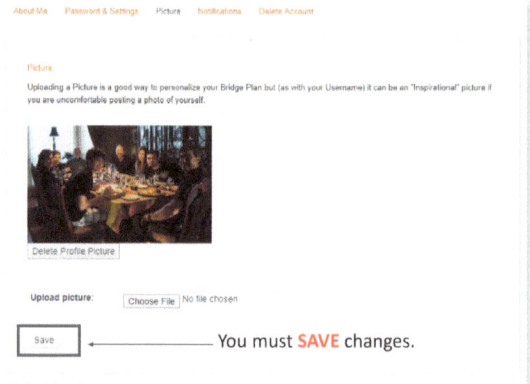

Notifications Page

Also in the Settings page, you can control which notifications and messages are emailed to you. Read these carefully. Then tick the boxes you want to use. Then click on Save.

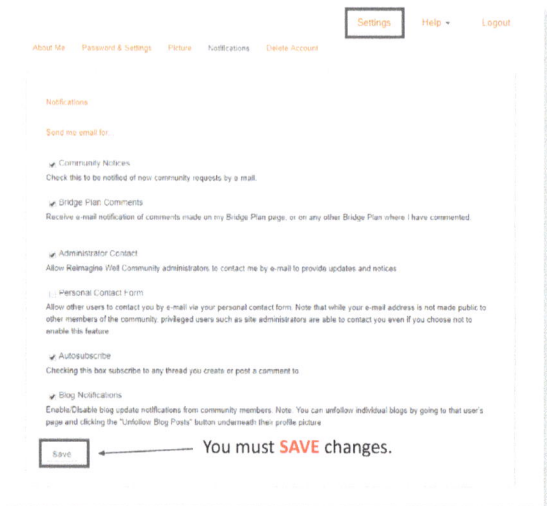

Deleting Accounts

If you wish to delete your account, you may do that in Settings. You will need your current password to do this.

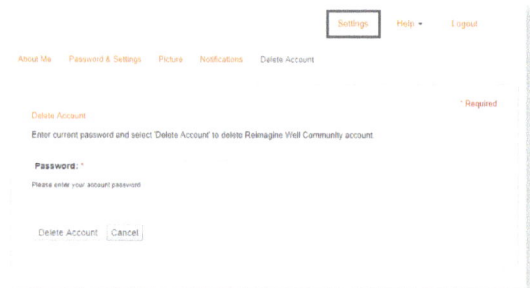

"As a long distance caregiver for my son, I love that I get notified about blogs here. And I can use the search box to find blogs that pertain to stuff my son is dealing with."

— AYA Caregiver/Dad

Caregivers: The Settings Area Is Helpful For You, Too

This is where you may arrange to interact with other caregivers, stay in touch with them, and share "Best Practices" in a private setting.

> "It is so important for the caregiver/spouse to be understanding. Jim is always saying: "I don't know what you see in me, but I am glad you do! I do not see anything less than what I married because of this."
>
> — AYA Caregiver/Wife

Your Landing Page

The My Bridge Plan is your landing page when you are logged in. Be sure to Bookmark this page. You can stayed logged in and always return to this page. Or if you logout, you will return to the Login page.

Setting Achievable Health Goals

Understanding That It Works In Phases

Your Bridge Plan allows you to divide your cancer journey into phases. And you set achievable health Goals for each phase. Whether you've just been diagnosed, or are moving from treatment into healing, Goals are important. Life seems to make more sense - and give us a purpose - when we have a Goal.

> "I have found the information here to be invaluable. Particularly the emphasis on goals… and the need for us to proactively deal with our disease."
>
> — AYA Cancer Patient, Age 29, Breast Cancer

Setting Achievable Health Goals For Each Phase

Goals are the heart of your Bridge Plan. Setting Goals establishes a vision of your future. Adding Goals to your Bridge Plan enables your support community to hold you accountable. Knowing they have your back will give you strength.

Add Goals that will move you toward your Survivorship. Whenever possible, make your Goals as clean, clear, specific, time-bound and measurable as you can. For example:

"Call my parents every weekend and see how they are doing."
"Fix my relationship with my boss before my next work review."

"Find new friends who enhance my life before summer."

"Sign up for yoga classes before the end of the month."

"Get my bicycle repaired and ride it for an hour on the weekends."

Here is a great blog on how to set achievable health goals. (https://www.reimaginewellcommunity.com/node/7623)

"My goal is to utilize my inner-strength and find comfort from my family, friends and medical team!"
— AYA Cancer Patient, Age 35, Prostate Cancer

Completing Goals

Setting achievable health goals, and completing them, will help you continue to feel like you are moving forward. When you complete a Goal, check the box that is beside it and watch your completion graph grow! Your community of friends can tell how you are doing, and can encourage you on in the Comment section.

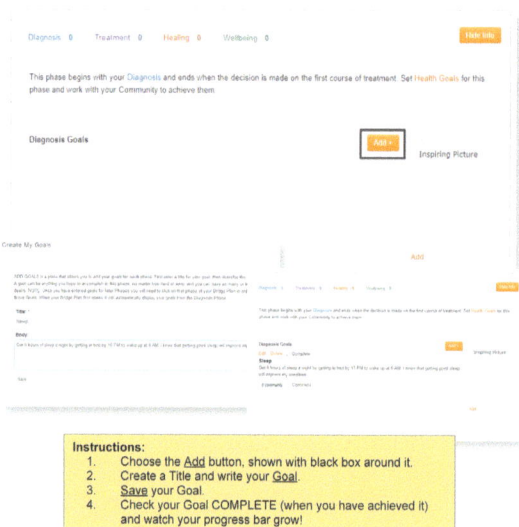

Instructions:
1. Choose the Add button, shown with black box around it.
2. Create a Title and write your Goal.
3. Save your Goal.
4. Check your Goal COMPLETE (when you have achieved it) and watch your progress bar grow!

"The support can save your life!! If you're confused and scared about your cancer diagnosis, then this is a good place to start on your journey to recovery."
— AYA Cancer Patient, Age 20, Brain Cancer

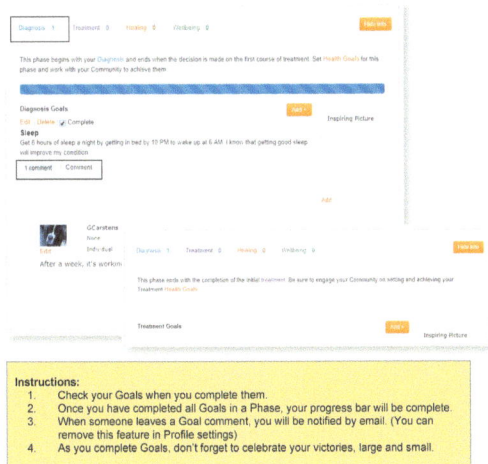

Instructions:
1. Check your Goals when you complete them.
2. Once you have completed all Goals in a Phase, your progress bar will be complete.
3. When someone leaves a Goal comment, you will be notified by email. (You can remove this feature in Profile settings)
4. As you complete Goals, don't forget to celebrate your victories, large and small.

Motivation Keeps You Going

It's not just the cheers and hoorays from the members of your community that will keep you going. You need other motivations to continue to move forward. Reward yourself with healthy treats, some new clothes, a book or music download you've always wanted. Think about that trip to Mexico or Hawaii that you've always dreamed about. Even something simple will do, like taking yourself out to a nice meal or walking through a beautiful park. Celebrate the good things and people in your life. Send your doctors a thank you note. Let your social worker know how you're doing. Thank friends who were there for you during your treatment. These things can be rewarding, and motivating, too!

What And Who Are Your Powerful Motivators?

Think about what else in life motivates you, excites you and gives you an emotional lift. It might be family, friends, loved ones, coworkers. Who were the people who rooted for you? Imagine their faces. Use those thoughts and memories to keep you going. Think of specific people, events, special occasions, vacations, your pets. The things that are your most powerful motivators are likely to be the things closest to you.

"Having something in your hands… a scrapbook with photos… it's such a motivational thing to have something you can feel and touch… to remind you 'this is why we're doing these things.'"
— AYA Caregiver/Grandmother

Gather Photos To Inspire You

Photos are a great way to share more about yourself in your Bridge Plan. They can remind you why you want to take control of your health journey. And they can inspire you to want to live to see tomorrow! Think about the photos you have on your desk at work, or on your laptop screen saver at school, or on your phone. Find the photos that make you laugh, smile and glad to be alive. Add your "Inspiring Pictures" to your Bridge Plan for you and your community members to see.

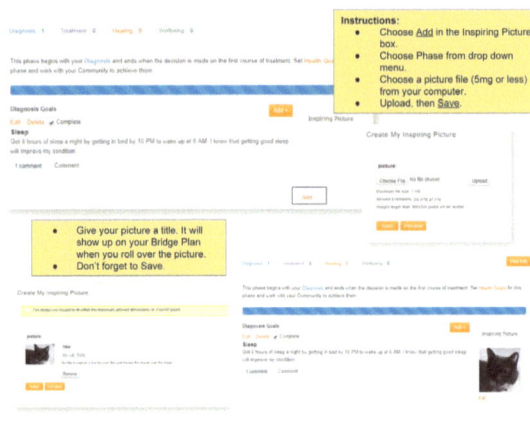

Learn to Tell Your Story

Sharing the story of your life, including your diagnosis, treatment, healing, wellbeing and Survivorship, is important. It's also a chronicle of what you've endured and what you've accomplished. Your story, when shared with others in your community, will help create a bond between you and them. You may not know it, but your story will help and inspire others. It will give them a glimpse into the truth of your life experiences. It may give them hope when they've run out of it.

Sharing your story, and commenting in a helpful way on the stories of others, is one more way you have of learning you are not alone. There are COMMENT buttons in several places on your Bridge Plan. These allow you and your community members to leave comments. And you will learn how to leave comments on their Bridge Plans, too

.

Bridge Plan

GCarstens
Date of Birth: 05/17/1990
US - California
Individual
None

Edit

Diagnosis 1   Treatment 0   Healing 0   Wellbeing 0   Hide Info

This phase begins with your Diagnosis and ends when the decision is made on the first course of treatment. Set Health Goals for this phase and work with your Community to achieve them

Diagnosis Goals   Add ▾   Inspiring Picture

Edit · Delete ✓ Complete
Sleep
Get 8 hours of sleep a night by getting in bed by 10 PM to wake up at 6 AM. I know that getting good sleep will improve my condition

1 comment   Comment

                              Share

                              Individual

Leave your comments here when you read my bridge Plan. I want to hear from you.

Share   LEAVE A COMMENT

"The paths we have travelled can be an inspiration for those who follow."
— AYA Cancer Patient, Age 32, Leukemia

Building Your Team

So you've begun your Bridge Plan at the phase of the journey which you are now in. You've posted information about yourself. You've written some achievable health goals. You've invited the people, and added photos, that motivate you. You've learned how to tell your story so other Bridge Builders - that is, other cancer patients and survivors like yourself who are a part of the Reimagine Well Support Community (http://www.reimaginewellcommunity.com/reimaginewell) - will read it, understand it, and relate to it. Maybe some of them have already begun to support you. And maybe some family members, friends or your members of your Care Team whom you've invited to be with you on your journey have written to you, too.

Always Surround Yourself With Love And Support

All of these people will become your Reimagine Well Community. You need people like that, who'll surround you with love and support. People who can understand and relate to what you've been through. Some of them will become your mentors, and some YOU will mentor. Just like real life.

Making a Safe, Supportive Community For Yourself

The Reimagine Well Support Communities are a place to gather your strongest allies. You can unite them to become an integrated part of the next step in your journey. In My Community, you can send invitations, and keep up with requests that you've sent and received. Everyone in your Community will automatically receive email updates when you post or comment on your blog.

> "Find a way to have fun… laugh and smile and bring people around you who'll allow you to laugh and smile!"
> — AYA Cancer Patient, Age 17, Osteosarcoma

Check Out The Suggested Community Members

Use the Suggested Community Members tool to connect with other Bridge Builders. These are people with whom you might have a lot in common. Take a moment to read about their cancer journey experiences and suggestions.

The first time you do this, give yourself a little time. Like any other new social platform, you may find yourself "falling down the rabbit hole."

A few hours later, you're gonna look up and say "These people get me!"

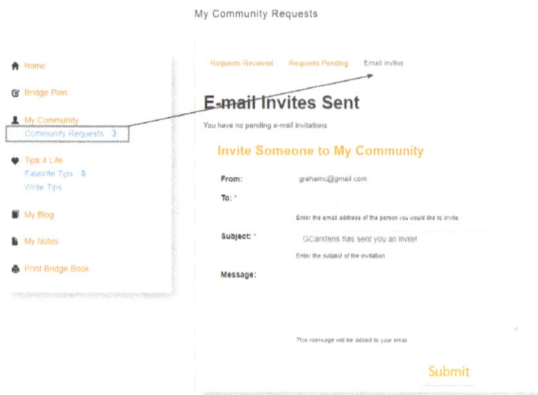

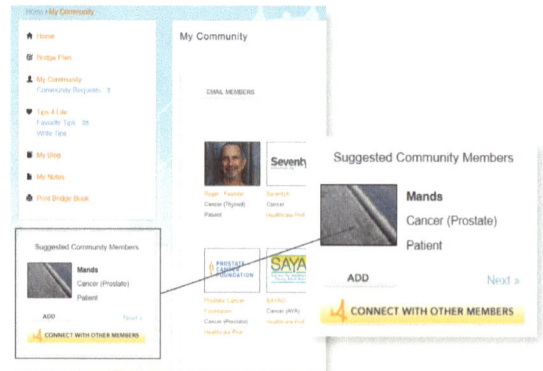

Find Your Tribe: The Benefits of Support Groups

You may be one of those who scoff or laugh at Support Groups. Give this one a try. Seriously. There is almost nothing better in the world than communicating with people who understand you and what you are going through. We call that "Finding Your Tribe."

There's another way to find Bridge Builders to add to your Community. It's the Connect With Other Members button. You can even filter other Bridge Builders by Illness, Condition, Phase, Role and Location. Go on. Find Your Tribe!

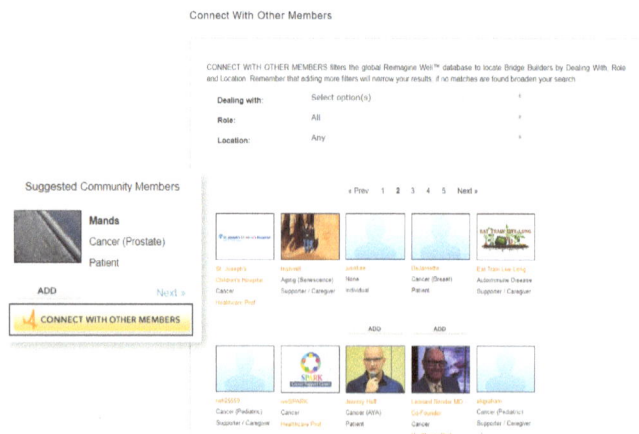

Other Support Organizations

When you first join, you may have only one or two Support Organizations in My Community. An easy way to find other Bridge Builders and Support Organizations is to visit their accounts. You will see all their members. And can send requests to them.

So that you know… accepting a community request is optional. Meaning it's not required by you, or by the person to whom you send the request.

My Blog and Commenting On Another's Blog

My Blog allows you to publicly share about your journey. Your Community will be told when you post a new blog; it's an easy way to co
mmunicate. Blog posts are searchable by our global community by tags, keywords, illness/condition. Blogs (and your other postings) are all reviewed by our medical staff and/or the National Cancer Institute before they are published . It may take up to 48 hours to see your blog in the feed. And if there are responses to your blog you feel are objectionable, you may remove them.

> "Beginning the process, telling my story, going back to explore, each step has been therapeutic!
> Through my blog, I give a voice to my journey and emotions."
> — AYA Cancer Patient, Age 34, Lung Cancer

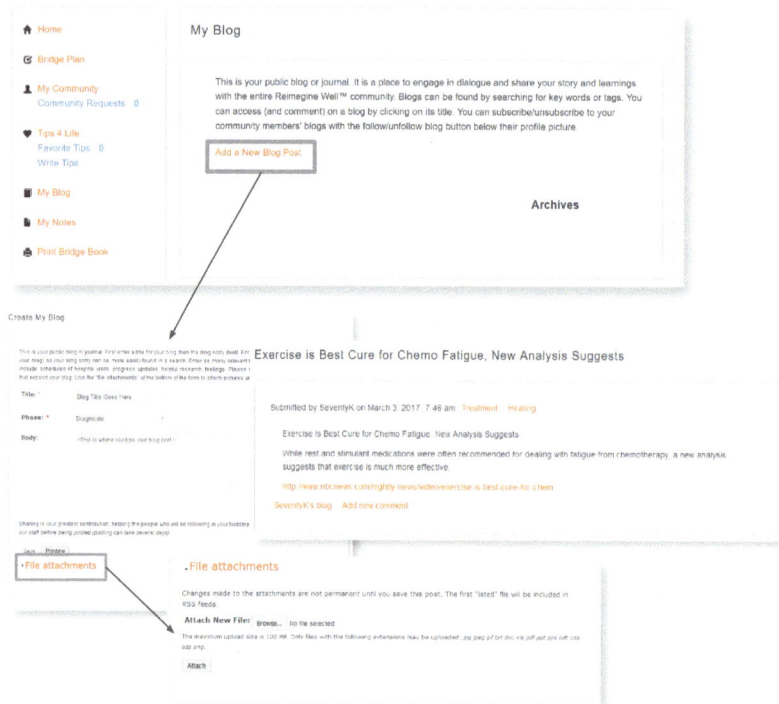

Instructions:
1. Choose Add a New Blog Post.
2. Pick a title, a Phase, add tags (keywords) and write your Blog post.
3. You can attach files to your Blog. Look for File Attachments below the text box and above the Save button.
4. Select Save and your Blog is created. (It will be reviewed before it is published and usually takes 24-48 hours)
5. Your Community members will be notified by email once it's published.
6. Community members can leave comments on your Blog post.
7. You can delete comments.
8. You can Edit or Delete your Blog.

To comment on another Bridge Builder's blog, look at the bottom of the blog. You'll find a Comment box. Enter a subject and your message. Then click the SAVE button. It will post but you will not see it immediately. It often takes a few moments for the comment to make its way through the administration function. The Blogger will receive an email notifying them about the comment, as will anyone who has left a comment.

"Coming Out" In Public, Social Media, Blogging

One more suggestion before we move on to other uses you can make of your Bridge Plan. "Coming out" to others about your illness, no matter what phase of it you are in, is a brave and often difficult thing to do.

Roger Holzberg, Reimagine Well's co-founder, and an adult cancer survivor, says it can be very complicated. Especially during diagnosis and treatment. There are so many people to keep up on what's currently happening. He recommends to newly diagnosed patients that they consider "what they expect" from those they tell during early phases.

For many of us, sharing every detail of your life on Facebook, Twitter, Instagram and other social media is just another part of daily life. That's not always true for members of older generations, who didn't grow up with social media.

However you feel about this, just remember whatever you decide to do publicly - let it all hang out or keep it close to the vest - understand that what you post about your Bridge Plan will be accessible to all of the people you accept into your community.

These people and you will share something in common. They will be your supporters and your allies. If you want to try out new thoughts or ideas about your illness with them first, it would be a great place to start. Then, as Dr. Sender says, "Go tell the world!"

Keeping Organized

Start With Medical Contact Information In My Notes

Use My Notes to keep track of contact information for nurses, doctors, physical therapists, nutritionists, etc. Under My Notes you can keep an organized record of other important information, too. This can include post-appointment summaries, details about medications you may be taking and the dosage, or advice from your medical professionals. After treatment is over, you can use your End of Treatment Summary to get this information.

PLEASE BE AWARE: In order to protect your medical information and insure its privacy, none of the medical information on this page is able to be shared publicly. If you'd like to share something with your community, you will need to enter it in your public blog.

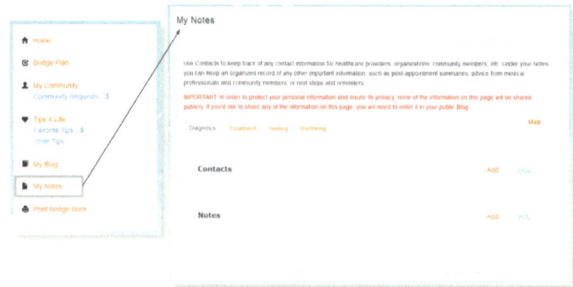

How To Record Post-Appointment Summaries, Medications and Dosages, Advice From Medical Professionals And Support Groups

Below are instructions on how to keep track of all the medical professionals with whom you interact. You can also record any and all medical notes here that you might need.

Again, the medical information here is always private. It can only be seen by you unless you print it out and show the printed paper to someone.

Tips 4 Life - From And For Others

Tips 4 Life is a global database of real world wisdom from regular people and healthcare professionals who have been just where you are now.

As you complete each phase of your cancer journey we strongly encourage you to leave behind Tips 4 Life for the people who are following in your footsteps.

Each time you want to check for new tips, click on My New Tips. That will open a window with the newest tips for the entire community.

To find the most relevant tips for you, select Filter Tips. After you use Filter Tips, My New Tips will open a window with the tips you have requested.

> "Folks learn because the authors can add tags and they are searchable!"
>
> — Cancer Patient, Age 38, Thyroid Cancer

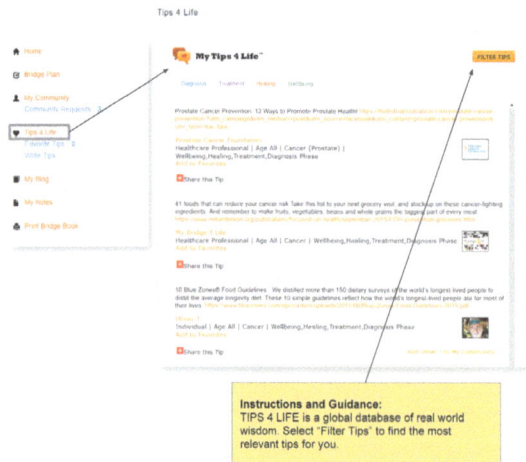

Instructions and Guidance:
TIPS 4 LIFE is a global database of real world wisdom. Select "Filter Tips" to find the most relevant tips for you.

You can begin by selecting an illness only, then clicking the Filter Tips button. After the window closes, click My New Tips to explore your tips. Selecting additional filters will narrow your tip results. R emember to save your favorites. If you'd like to gain deeper knowledge about a tip from your favorites, click on the Bridge Builder's name to join their community. That way you can contact them directly with questions about their tip.

As you work through this section of the Bridge Plan, you'll find instructions about how to select your Favorite Tips, contact other Bridge Builders, write tips of your own and how to search through other Tips 4 Life and Blogs. In the Help section, there is also a full start-up guide with "Best Practices" available to download if necessary.

Use Your Bridge Plan Journal

You can keep a private journal of your own thoughts and experiences. You may also record ideas and future suggestions for others who will follow in your path. Remember that someday your writing will be helpful to someone else.

Print Your Bridge Book - Chronicle Of Your Journey

You can also print out your Bridge Book. We encourage all Bridge Builders to print a copy of their Bridge Book after each phase of their journey. You should bring it to any meetings with your Care Team. Your printed Bridge Book becomes a chronicle of your journey, from Diagnosis through Treatment, Healing, and on to Wellbeing.

Healing and Moving Forward

As Dr. Sender said at the beginning of this Learn Guide: "You have to become empowered to ask the right questions, and to find the right questions to get the information you need." In other words, Knowledge Is Power.

Resources For Healing and Moving Forward

There are many resources for your wellbeing and your Survivorship. This Learn Guide is full of links to reputable and reliable organizations whom you can trust, specifically the National Institutes of Health (https://www.nih.gov/), the National Cancer Institute (https://www.cancer.gov/) and the American Cancer Society (https://www.cancer.org/). You should feel free to roam around their websites, along with the links below.

TO LEARN MORE

NCI Office of Survivorship - Resources: https://cancercontrol.cancer.gov/ocs/resources/survivors.html

Cancer Survivors Managing Their Health: https://www.cancer.org/latest-news/new-website-to-help-cancer-survivors-manage-health.html

Cancer Survivorship Research: http://bit.ly/2wqVeQf

Coping With Cancer Survivorship: https://www.cancer.gov/about-cancer/coping/survivorship

NCI - A Tough Transition to Cancer Survivorship: https://www.cancer.gov/about-cancer/coping/research/survivorship-plans

Getting Mentored

Do you still feel as if you might need a mentor? Someone to help you through whatever phase you are in now? There are many places where you can find someone to talk to, and perhaps even spend some time with. These services do exist. As the expression goes: help is just a phone call away. You'll find a list of links to these services below.

Being A Mentor

Mentoring is a process by which you share your experiences with another cancer patient. Often this is a patient who is experiencing what you have already gone through. By doing this, you empower them. You give them hope. And you strengthen them for what lies ahead. You can mentor other patients by volunteering at the hospital where you were treated, or your own local hospital. You can help in an online community or by phone.

"Every cancer survivor is a researcher. As you communicate your treatment and what you have been through, your doctors will continue to learn and use this knowledge to treat the patients who follow you. So, don't stop communicating – your doctors always learn and adapt treatment based on the knowledge that they gain from you!"

— Lilibeth Torno, M.D.

TO LEARN MORE

Organizations & Resources to Support Young Cancer Patients: https://www.cancer.gov/types/aya

4th Angel – Patient & Caregiver Mentoring Program: http://www.4thangel.org/

Cancer Connects Volunteer Mentor Program: http://www.cancerconnects.org/volunteerMentorProgram

Imerman Angels: http://imermanangels.org/

The Future

As we told you at the beginning of this Learn Guide, stop and take a breath. Let it out, long and slow. Look around you. Look behind you. Look forward.

That's the way you are heading now. Straight into your New Normal.

Cancer has a way of doing that to people. It makes them see, hear and feel what is really important. What matters. What counts.

A walk down a country road in the fall, as the leaves are glowing a bright red and yellow. A July 4th dinner with your family where everyone gets along. Watching the sun set over the ocean, a lake, or even a glacier.

Getting together with friends that you love, and who love you back. Hugging those friends and telling them "Thank you for being there for me." And then turning around and being there for them when they need you.

Life, it is said, can be wonderful, awful, strange, funny and familiar, all at the same time. It can also be hard and frustrating, glorious and awesome.

If you're reading this, you're still here.
That's what is important.
That's what matters.
That's what counts.

You have been deepened, broadened and strengthened by your cancer journey. You've grown. You're a different person now. And you're not alone.

Take one more deep breath.

Then start walking straight into your well-earned Survivorship.

"Keep healthy. Keep your spirit up. Live every day to the fullest!"
— AYA Cancer Patient, Age 30, Lymphoma

From Team Reimagine Well

"I've been involved with pediatric cancers, adolescents, and young adults for nearly 30 years. The thing I want to say to a patient who has just completed their treatment is, firstly, congratulations and, secondly, well done. What we need to talk about now is how we get you to your new normal, how we get you to adulthood, how we understand all the consequences of the therapy that you've been through, and how we make sure that you truly have wellness going forward."

— Leonard Sender, M.D.

"I am a three time AYA cancer survivor. I had osteogenic sarcoma when I was 15, with two relapses, and I had ovarian cancer when I was 38. I hope that by seeing me "Get Busy Living", patients have hope that it is possible to survive and thrive after cancer. It's also very important for me to help educate patients to become strong survivors."

— Jenee Areeckal, MSW, LCSW

"I'm a cancer specialist, and I take care of childhood cancer survivors.
The most important thing I would say to anyone who just finished therapy is congratulations.
This is a major achievement in your cancer journey."

— Lilibeth Torno, M.D.

"This is the time to nourish and nurture yourself. Take advantage of the resources that are available to help you make the best choices. When it comes to food and nutrition, reach out to a registered dietitian nutritionist. You will be in the hands of an expert who is trained to help you deal with your journey to Wellbeing and Survivorship."

— Jocelyn Harrison, MPH, RN

"This is what your Bridge Plan is designed for: To move you from diagnosis to wellbeing by setting achievable health goals in each phase. And then to enable and encourage mentoring and sharing wisdom.
For me, it was nearly a year post-surgery before I was really ready to open up about the experience and share...
There will come a time when you look back on this with perspective and newfound knowledge.
The knowledge you share eases the journey for those following in your footsteps."

— Roger Holzberg, Cancer Survivor and Co-Founder Of Reimagine Well

NOTES

Learn Guide Authors

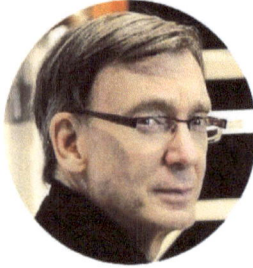

Martin Casella

Martin is an award-winning educator, playwright and screenwriter. He has taught writing at the California Institute of the Arts and at the Harvey Milk School, a NYC public high school with a focus on At Risk and LGBTQ students. At HMHS he created a writing program where teens learned to shape their life stories. The "What's Your Story" program now serves as a fundraising tool for the HMHS Student College Scholarship Fund. Martin has also written for Steven Spielberg, Kerry Washington, Lasse Hallstrom, Anthony Edwards, Whoopi Goldberg, John Milius, HBO, Disney, Universal, Warner Brothers and Paulist Productions. Among the writing awards he has won or been nominated for are The New York International Fringe Festival Overall Excellence Award for Playwriting (twice); the New York Outer Critics Circle for Best New Off-Broadway Musical; two GLAAD Award nominations for Outstanding New Play and Best New Off-Broadway Musical, and the LA WEEKLY Outstanding New Play Award. Martin's plays are published by Samuel French and been performed worldwide. He has written for Opera News, and his interactive writing credits include Steven Spielberg's Director's Chair.

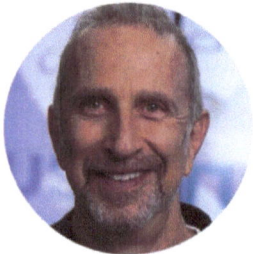

Roger Holzberg

Roger is the founder of My Bridge for Life™ and served as the first (consulting) Creative Director for the National Cancer Institute (NCI) where he led a multi-discipline Team to concept and build NCI's vision of how to educate patients, researchers and healthcare professionals. The "evolution" of cancer.gov, the NCI Facebook, Twitter, and YouTube networks are all projects that his creative team took from concept through launch. Previously, Roger spent 12 years as an award-winning Creative Director / Vice President at Walt Disney Imagineering where he had the opportunity to lead the creative development for a broad portfolio of projects ranging from PlayStation® games to theme park icons and several Disney World Celebrations; from mass audience interactive experiences and rides; to the MMOG Virtual Magic Kingdom. In "classic media," Roger has written and directed feature films and television, but is genuinely proud of researching and writing "The Living Sea" (Academy Award nomination for best documentary – Imax). Personally, Roger is a proud father; a 14+ year cancer survivor; and a competitive triathlete (3 events yearly), using the sport to raise research dollars for causes he supports.

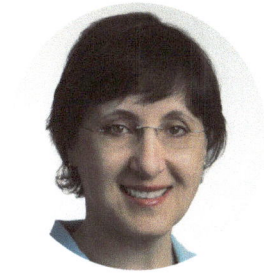

Adele Sender

Adele has developed clinical systems for healthcare software for complex chemotherapy regimens for diseases including HIV/AIDS and leukemia, and designed training modules for technology resource poor environments as well as expert systems. She has a BS in Physical Therapy, and serves on both education and patient advocacy boards.

If you, or someone you love, has been diagnosed with cancer Reimagine Well's Learn Guides are designed to guide you from diagnosis to wellbeing. We also provide a (private and safe) support community to connect with, where you can learn from the survivors and caregivers who have gone before you.

To learn more about our services, or to contact us directly, visit www.reimaginewell.com.

Our Videos & eBooks are not substitutes or replacements for your health-care providers. They are designed to provide education and focus and help you optimize the care plan you elect to pursue with your doctor.

If you are having a medical emergency of any kind, call your doctor, 911, or emergency services immediately.

www.ingramcontent.com/pod-product-compliance
Lightning Source LLC
Chambersburg PA
CBHW060801270326
41926CB00002B/56